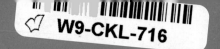
W9-CKL-716

THE HEALTH IMPACT ASSESSMENT
OF DEVELOPMENT
PROJECTS

M H BIRLEY

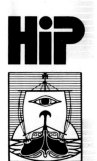

The Health Impact Programme
Liverpool School of Tropical Medicine
Pembroke Place
Liverpool L3 5QA

LONDON: HMSO

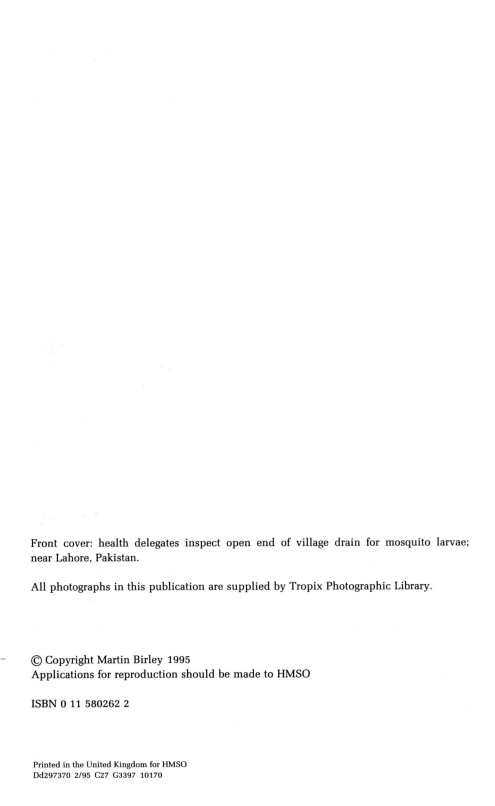

Front cover: health delegates inspect open end of village drain for mosquito larvae; near Lahore, Pakistan.

All photographs in this publication are supplied by Tropix Photographic Library.

© Copyright Martin Birley 1995
Applications for reproduction should be made to HMSO

ISBN 0 11 580262 2

Printed in the United Kingdom for HMSO
Dd297370 2/95 C27 G3397 10170

FOREWORD

I am delighted to have been asked to write a foreword to this important milestone linking environment, health and development. These are issues of global concern. Although expressed in the language of a different age, it was that concern which underwrote the establishment of the Liverpool School of Tropical Medicine and its sister institutions during the last century. At that time we were barely at the beginning of our journey in medical research. A voyage that has now established the cause of so many common diseases. As the School draws towards its centenary, we seek new ways to apply that knowledge through teaching and technical assistance.

In 1990 the Overseas Development Administration agreed to support a work programme concerned with the health impact of development projects. This programme showed considerable foresight. Concern about the impact of development on the environment and on human health has continued to grow. The theme was set for the global community in the 21st century by the United Nations Conference on Environment and Development: the goal is a healthy people, living in a healthy and sustainable environment. Many countries have adopted, or are beginning to adopt, development planning policies which share that aim. This book will be invaluable to any professional seeking to apply such a policy – and particularly those with little experience of integrating human health.

Martin Birley is ably qualified to undertake this multi-disciplinary task. Following a first class honours degree in engineering science he turned his attention to biology. His research used mathematics and computer modelling to analyse agricultural and, later, medical pest populations. From there he moved to environmental management for vector control. He is a member of the Joint WHO/FAO/UNEP/UNCHS Panel of Experts in Environmental Management. Martin established the basis for this present work by examining the vector-borne diseases associated with water resource development. During the course of researching Health Impact Assessment he has worked with the World Health Organisation, the Food and Agriculture Organisation and the Asian Development Bank. He has taken part in workshops, seminars and training courses in many developing countries. Martin has also researched methods of inter-disciplinary communication and the use of hypertext technology as a presentation tool. Consequently, this book is one of the first outputs from the School to be published in both paper and electronic format. It will fill a significant gap in the Environmental Impact Assessment literature.

DH Molyneux, MA PhD DSc Cbiol FIBiol
Director, Liverpool School of Tropical Medicine
13 December, 1994

PREFACE

Governments and international agencies invest large sums on development projects in energy, agriculture, industry and other sectors. The environmental impact of these projects is frequently assessed. But it is the experience of many health professionals that the health impact receives too little attention. This book has been written to redress that balance.

Health Impact Assessment is a young and growing field of endeavour. During the course of preparation for this book three relevant publications have been issued by WHO that review linkages between health, environment and development. The Asian Development Bank have issued guidelines and the Australian government have produced a national framework. Reviews are a necessary but not a sufficient condition for health impact assessment. They are necessary because a process of classification provides the first step towards prediction: what has happened on an existing project is the best predictor of what could happen on a future project. They are not sufficient because impact assessment must take place within a framework in which donors, governments, planning officers, the general public and independent consultants are all informed of their role. The framework should include an agreed set of formal procedures for assessing and managing the health impacts of development projects. Such procedures have yet to be widely agreed. Procedures for industrial projects have developed further in response to the needs of industrialised economies and there is a specialist literature on that theme which we do not cover. The primary focus for this book is the rural sector and the rural poor. We follow them into their new urban environments and draw attention to the health hazards that they face in poorly regulated industries and settlements.

This book connects reviews and procedures and provides a readily accessible catalogue of health/development linkages. It is intended for a wide audience of students and practitioners both within the health sector and within fields concerned with environment or development. It advocates the need for health impacts to receive more attention within the existing framework of Environmental Impact Assessment. Many problems remain unanswered and there is much scope for further work.

Dr Martin H Birley
Health Impact Programme Manager

ACKNOWLEDGEMENTS

I would like to acknowledge the valuable suggestions, comments and contributions to the review supplied by the following: Dr RW Ashford, Mr R Bos, Ms TE Butler, Ms CR McConnell, Mr S Connor, Dr JBS Coulter, Dr AK Cassells, Mr D Curran, Mr WTS Gould, Dr AA Hassan, Professor RG Hendrickse, Dr JM Jewsbury, Ms N Kernighan, Professor WW Macdonald, Dr C Macpherson, Dr SM Maxwell, Professor RH Meakins, Dr IS Narula, Dr CA Pearson, Ms GL Peralta, Mr ER Potts, Dr JE Price, Dr MW Service, Dr DH Smith, Dr AW Smith, Dr H Townson, Dr RD Ward, Dr GB White, Dr GB Wyatt, Dr A Zwi. Many thanks to our research assistant, Ms TE Butler, who painstakingly checked copy and references. Mr IK Parry helped with reference management, formatting, printing and related computer skills. Ms T Hewitt provided invaluable secretarial support. Ms B Lewis sub-edited the copy.

Part of the review material was incorporated in the Asian Development Bank Paper No. 11 entitled "Guidelines for the Health Impact of Development Projects", during 1992. Preparation of that document, with co-author Ms GL Peralta, was invaluable for understanding the institutional procedures listed in chapter 1. We are grateful to the ADB for permission to use that material.

The San Serriffe exercise was modified from one prepared in collaboration with Professor CE Engel for use in a joint PEEM/DBL training course in Zimbabwe. We thank Guardian Newspapers Ltd for permission to use the imaginary country name San Serriffe which they created.

The preparation of this book was funded by the Health and Population Division of the Overseas Development Administration, as part of a five year work programme at the Liverpool School of Tropical Medicine. It draws on the accumulated experiences of many colleagues at the Liverpool School of Tropical Medicine and at leading institutions in Europe and the Tropics. It was facilitated by the invaluable trust, support and encouragement provided, first, by the Dean, Professor RG Hendrickse, and later by the Director, Professor DH Molyneux. Finally, I acknowledge my family, Veronica, Roland and Lawrence all of whom must suffer my frequent absence. Veronica's support and interest has been invaluable.

The views and statements presented in this book are the responsibility of the author alone and do not necessarily reflect those of any other individual or organization.

ABBREVIATIONS

dB	decibels. Units of measurement of sound
dBA	decibel level reaching the ear from external sound
DBL	Danish Bilharziasis Laboratory
EC	European Community
EIA	Environmental Impact Assessment
FAO	Food and Agriculture Organization
GNP	Gross National Product
ha	hectare
HIA	Health Impact Assessment
HIV	Human Immunodeficiency Virus
HYV	High Yielding Varieties
IHE	Initial Health Examination
IPM	Integrated Pest Management
IRRI	International Rice Research Institute
JE	Japanese Encephalitis
km	kilometre
μg	microgram
m	metre
M	million
OHS	Occupational Health and Safety
PEEM	The joint WHO/FAO/UNEP/UNCHS Panel of Experts on Environmental Management for vector control
PNG	Papua New Guinea
STD	Sexually Transmitted Disease
TB	tuberculosis
TOR	Terms of Reference
ULV	Ultra Low Volume
uv-B	ultraviolet-B radiation
WHO	World Health Organization

CONTENTS

chapter 1

1   WHY APPRAISE HEALTH IMPACT?

The sustainability of development can only be ensured if the full range of potential impacts are appraised in a timely fashion and actions proceed from that appraisal.

The potential impacts of development are numerous and cut across many specialist concerns. Most development projects, from whatever sector, are expected to have a beneficial effect on human health by increasing the resources available for food, education, employment, water supplies, sanitation, and health services. If the project is in the health sector the health benefit is the intended objective. This book is concerned exclusively with the non-health sectors, in which health impacts are an indirect consequence of the development.

Sometimes the indirect impacts include unexpected negative effects on health. Many of these can be avoided by careful planning. Adverse health impacts are most likely to affect the most vulnerable social groups. The poor, ethnic and religious minorities, women, children and the elderly may be at especially increased risk; they tend to have poorer access to resources or lack the political power which may be necessary to promote their interests. This may serve to amplify the overall adverse effect. Such impacts reduce the social and economic benefits expected from the development and transfer hidden costs to the health sector.

Health appraisal offers an opportunity to identify health hazards in advance. Often only minor actions may be required to safeguard health. The actions may vary from ensuring that the health authorities are informed of development plans, to specific requests for major planning changes, such as settlement siting. In addition, the analysis of health risk provides an opportunity to incorporate health promoting activities in the development project.

2   ENVIRONMENTAL IMPACT ASSESSMENT

Many countries have now recognised the need to legislate and establish procedures to protect the natural environment from over-exploitation. Concerns range from the discharge of damaging chemicals to the loss of archaeological heritage. The usual procedure is as follows.

An Environmental Protection Agency, Council or Division is established to license and monitor new developments. The licensing arrangements involve the preparation of an environmental impact statement by the project proponent. Subsidiary activities include a project screening procedure to prevent planning delays and establish priorities and a scoping procedure to ensure that all interested parties are consulted and all aspects of the impact are included. The central activity is the Environmental Impact Assessment. This is commissioned from a qualified consultant who works to detailed terms of reference. The assessment is intended to identify and predict the impact of the project on the biogeographical environment and on people's health and well-being and to interpret and communicate information about the impacts.

It is the experience of many professionals that the health component receives too little attention, especially within developing countries. This book has been written to redress that balance. It does not propose a separate and parallel procedure for health impact assessment. Rather, it proposes to incorporate health impact assessment within environmental impact assessment. The procedures described are consistent with those currently used to assess the biogeographical environment. They have been modified as necessary to encompass health.

3   AUDIENCE

This book has been written with several different groups of readers in mind. These include:

◆ Students of environmental science for whom an introduction to health and development issues would be relevant.

◆ Students of development studies and development project planning.

◆ Managers of environmental protection agencies in developing countries who ensure that national standards are maintained prior to granting a licence for development.

◆ Project planning managers in donor agencies and aid organisations. Such managers are not, themselves, health specialists. They are frequently economists, agriculturalists or engineers. Nevertheless, they must decide when a health impact assessment is required, commission a study and appraise the study report.

◆ Consultants who are assigned to undertake health impact assessment. Such assignments are frequently subsumed under an environmental impact assessment. The consultants are often generalists within the fields of ecology, environment or health.

◆ Health specialists who are interested in learning about development planning or impact assessment procedures.

◆ Health specialists who want a readily accessible list of the health hazards associated with development projects.

4   REVIEWS OF HEALTH IMPACT

There are already several books from the World Health Organization that describe or review the potential health impacts of development projects and environmental change[1,2,3]. Such reviews are necessarily incomplete. We have summarized from them and added new material for our own review. Reviews themselves serve only to highlight the problem. We seek to provide an operational procedure with which to appraise health impact. One component of the procedure is a classification scheme. Classification is a crucial step in prediction. Projects classified as similar at the outset are likely to share the same impacts. Therefore, our review is systematically classified. We use a scheme which focuses on the sector of the economy in which the development project is being undertaken. We also classify the range of health problems into simple categories.

When impacts have been identified, health risk management measures can be included in project plans and operation in order to reduce the risk and to minimise the extent of the adverse consequences.

5   HOW TO ASSESS HEALTH IMPACT

The proposed procedure for assessing health impacts is adapted from one that we prepared for the Asian Development Bank[4]. The main steps in health impact assessment are:

◆   Identification of health hazards;

◆   Interpretation as health risks;

◆   Management of health risks.

The operational procedures required by a regulating agency to achieve these steps are:

◆   Initial screening of the project for health hazards;

◆   Initial health examination, or rapid appraisal;

◆   Health impact assessment;

◆   Proposals for health risk management.

The initial screening process identifies the health hazards normally associated with the kind of development project in the specified location. For example, schistosomiasis is a health hazard for an irrigation project in Tanzania. This step will normally be carried out by the project officer.

The initial health examination (IHE), or rapid appraisal, uses existing information to interpret the health hazard as a health risk. It will normally be carried out by an officer responsible for impact assessment. The distinction between a health hazard and a health risk is important and is discussed below. At the end of this step, the project receives a health impact classification. The classification may indicate the need for a full health impact assessment.

A full health impact assessment (HIA) is carried out by a specialist consultant according to terms of reference drawn up by a project manager. It involves detailed field studies and is a more rigorous, expensive and specific form of assessment.

These are the same procedures used by many donor agencies for environmental impact assessment. The first two steps are necessary in order to ensure that development projects are not delayed unnecessarily by lengthy or expensive investigations.

Health risk management consists of modifications to project plans, operations or maintenance. It includes both health safeguards and mitigation measures. Project monitoring and health surveillance are also required.

6   WHEN TO ASSESS HEALTH IMPACT

Where significant health risks are attributable to the project, it may be appropriate to manage the health risks by designing health safeguards and mitigation measures. These measures must be incorporated in project plans,

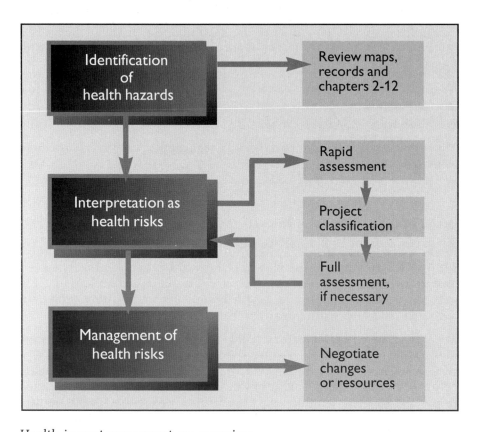

Health impact assessment, an overview

operations and maintenance schedules. Experience suggests that in order for project plans to be modified, negotiations must begin at a very early stage in the project cycle. This is usually referred to as the pre-feasibility stage. After this stage the investment in engineering design is considerable and so are the costs of modification. It follows that impact assessments must take place at the pre-feasibility stage and that they should be as rapid as possible. There is rarely an opportunity for a rigorous scientific study.

The project cycle and the process of negotiation with application to irrigation and dam projects has been described by Tiffen[5].

Health impact studies also form part of the *ex-post* project evaluation. Lessons may be learnt that can influence future planning and appraisal.

7 SCOPE OF BOOK

The scope of development projects considered in this book is limited to project rather than programme aid. The many health impacts of macroeconomic policies are reviewed in a recent World Health Organization/World Bank publication[3]. Macroeconomic policies such as structural adjustment, commodity pricing, import restrictions, direct food aid, debt servicing, farm subsidies, removal of food subsidies, taxation on alcohol and tobacco products, have major impacts on food production, food security, malnutrition and health status. By contrast, this book focuses on project aid where there is a change in the physical environment. When people change the physical environment, health impact assessment is a component of environmental impact assessment. Table 1 summarizes the main development sectors considered.

Health sector projects themselves will not be discussed as it is assumed that their health impacts will be assessed by health specialists. Health sector

TABLE I The main development sectors

Development Sector	Examples
Transport and Communication	Road construction, bus services
Mining	Opencast, tin, coal, gold, asbestos
Energy	Dams and hydropower, thermal
Renewable Natural Resources	Agriculture, irrigation, fisheries, forestry, livestock
Public Services	Low cost housing, resettlement, water supply
Manufacture and Trade	Industrial production, tourism

projects can have negative health impacts. For example, health workers are exposed to a range of occupational health hazards. However, we do include hospital waste disposal and vector control by insecticides.

A third group of projects concern education and training, or human resource development. The possible indirect health benefits are outside the scope of this book.

Finally, the focus of our method is rural/natural resource development rather than urban/industrial projects. There is already a specialist literature on the health hazards of industrial development. This literature is especially concerned with the regulation of emissions and occupational safety. We are primarily concerned about the rural poor. We follow them into their new urban environment and draw attention to the health hazards that they face in poorly regulated industries and settlements.

8   TYPES OF HEALTH HAZARD

A health hazard has a potential to cause disease or infirmity. The health risk indicates the extent to which the potential is realised. For example, malaria is a major health hazard in the tropics and sub-tropics. However, in some localities the risk may be small because there are few mosquitoes capable of transmitting the infection or the temperature is too low.

Health hazards may be further ranked according to the magnitude of their consequences. A major consequence would include multiple loss of life and chronic disability. A moderate consequence would include some loss of life and extensive temporary disability. A project which had a high risk of a major hazard would be unacceptable. A minor hazard of low risk may be unimportant. The importance attached to hazards and risks is culturally and politically determined and outside the scope of this discussion[6,7].

Although health must be viewed in its totality, for the purposes of impact assessment it is necessary to consider specific hazards and their components. The process of assessment consists of ranking these as likely to increase or decrease in magnitude as a result of the development intervention. The economic cost of the change in health hazard may be viewed as the additional cost of restoring to their previous state of health all the individuals who succumb to the additional hazard, plus the loss of production. That costing is the subject of current research by the Liverpool Health Impact Programme.

It is convenient to divide the health hazards associated with development projects into five main categories, listed in Table 2.

TABLE 2 Types of health hazard

Health hazard	Examples and causes
Communicable disease	Malaria, diarrhoea, respiratory infection
Non-communicable disease	Poisoning, pollution, dust
Malnutrition	Reduced subsistence foods (inadequate food intake or micronutrient deficiencies)
Injury	Traffic crashes and collisions, occupational injury, violence
Mental disorder	Substance abuse, stress

8.1 COMMUNICABLE DISEASE

Communicable diseases require infectious agents which multiply in the host. They may be transmitted in air, water, food, dust, blood products, body fluids, faeces, soil and insect bite. In relation to development projects, they may be broadly sub-divided as follows:

◆ Diseases exacerbated by poor living conditions (eg. *scabies, meningitis, respiratory infection*).

◆ Diseases of poor water supply and sanitation (eg. *diarrhoea, cholera, typhoid, hookworm, hepatitis*).

◆ Sexually transmitted diseases (eg. *HIV, gonorrhoea*).

◆ Vector-borne diseases (eg. *malaria, schistosomiasis*).

◆ Zoonoses (eg. *pig tapeworm infection*).

The most common childhood killers include diarrhoea, respiratory infection, measles and malaria.

The infectious agents are distributed widely, but patchily, in the environment. Control may involve many small environmental modifications. Once an infection is introduced to a new community it may spread explosively from infected to uninfected people. Measles infection is an example.

8.2 NON-COMMUNICABLE DISEASE

The non-communicable diseases include those which result from the ingestion, absorption or inhalation of chemicals and certain minerals. These may be associated with pollution and poor occupational safety. They may cause organic damage. For example, dust inhalation damages the lungs. Other diseases result from stress.

The vulnerability of the community to the health impact of pollution is increased by malnutrition, communicable disease and human behaviour. In addition, pollution may increase susceptibility to communicable disease.

Some non-communicable diseases are the result of exposure to non-biological effluent produced at well-defined point sources.

Control may involve effluent reduction. For example, emissions from a factory chimney have a single, controllable, source.

EXAMPLES

◆ Agro-chemicals are often stored in the home and children play with empty, but contaminated, containers.

◆ Dust induced lung disease can facilitate infection with tuberculosis.

8.3   MALNUTRITION

All development projects are likely to have an impact on the food security and nutritional status of people living within (and possibly outside) the project area. Some agricultural projects will have improvements in food security as their specific objective. Other projects, such as mining, rural water supply and road construction, can have an impact on nutrition through a variety of indirect and possibly unplanned mechanisms. These include food production, food availability, workload, infection and feeding practices. They are described in more detail in later chapters.

Under-nourished people are more susceptible to communicable disease. The disease, in turn, may reduce their ability to assimilate whatever food is available.

The effects of malnutrition include less than average weight or height, blindness, cretinism, anaemia and poor skin conditions. Especially vulnerable groups include young children and pregnant or lactating women. The household often cannot be treated as a unit when considering access to adequate food.

The health impact assessment should determine whether all the communities associated with the project will have physical and economic access to adequate food at all times.

EXAMPLE

◆ New kinds of crops may require more weeding by women who then wean their babies earlier.

8.4   INJURY

Exposure to new technologies, poor working practices, poor dwelling design, improper use of machinery and poor machinery maintenance lead to acute or chronic injury. Injuries are often referred to as accidents and this implies that they cannot be prevented. However, most injury is the result of inappropriate human behaviour and poor management.

Wounds provide a route of entry for infectious agents. Sick individuals may operate machinery in a dangerous manner, increasing their vulnerability to further injury. Injured people are less productive and may suffer from malnutrition. Injuries may lead to disability which may be temporary or permanent.

Low safety standards are common in many countries. Occupational health and safety data is frequently unavailable. Development often involves construction. Labour is often sub-contracted to the lowest bidder who operates without regard for health, safety or good employment practice.

Disruption of traditional working and social patterns plus uneven patterns of development, may induce violent behaviour which causes injury.

EXAMPLE

◆   Eye damage occurs in quarrying, hearing damage occurs in weaving factories, burns and scalds occur in metal processing. Burns and scalds may also follow the introduction of wood replacement cooking stoves.

8.5   MENTAL DISORDER

Mental disorder may be associated with the stress of new ways of living and the disruption of long established communities. Associated problems include alcoholism, suicide, violence, eating disorders, heart disease and raised blood pressure. There is relatively little information about the prevalence of mental disorder in developing countries or the association with development projects[8].

8.6   INTERACTIONS BETWEEN HEALTH AND DEVELOPMENT

'A development path that combines growth with reduced vulnerability is more sustainable than one that does not[9].'

Although good health is not sufficient in itself, healthy people are believed to be more able to contribute positively to their own economic development, more willing to accept innovation, more careful and more able to look after each other[10]. They may be more likely to see themselves, and be seen by others, as the beneficiaries of development rather than its victims.

Health is associated with broader economic and demographic trends. Chronically sick populations have a lower economic output and less food may be produced or consumed. Poorer nutrition, in turn, increases susceptibility to disease and there is a downward spiral. Demographic trends are affected as more children may be required to compensate for those that are lost.

For a broader discussion see "Our Planet, Our Health, Report of the WHO Commission on Health and Environment"[1]. See also "Health Dimensions of Economic Reform"[2].

8.7   ASSOCIATION OF HEALTH HAZARD AND PROJECT STAGE

Some health hazards become health risks as soon as the community is exposed. This may occur while the community is in transition during the project construction phase. Health risk management should already be in operation. Other health hazards have a considerable latent period, ten years or longer, before they become apparent at the community level. Table 3 provides some examples. The health impact assessment must consider the whole life of the project.

TABLE 3   Examples of health problems with slow and fast onset

Health categories	Slow onset	Fast onset
Communicable disease	Filariasis, schistosomiasis, hookworm, ascariasis, tuberculosis	Malaria, enteric infections, dengue, meningitis, pneumonia
Non-communicable disease	Dust induced lung disease, chronic poisoning, cancers	Acute poisoning
Malnutrition	Goitre, blindness, stunting	Wasting
Injury	White finger, hearing and sight loss, posture	Trauma (crushing, breaking, wounding), burns, eye damage

Each stage of the project cycle provides opportunities to safeguard health. For example:

◆   Location affects exposure to vector-borne disease.

◆   Design affects abundance of vector breeding sites.

◆   Construction may mix communities in ways that favour a range of communicable disease transmission.

◆   Operation introduces conditions for occupational health risks.

See also Health Risk Management, section 15.

9   EXAMPLES OF HEALTH/DEVELOPMENT LINKAGES

Figure 1 illustrates some of the linkages between health and development. These linkages are explained below. More details are provided in later chapters of this book.

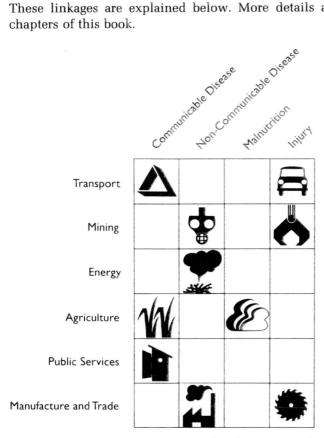

Figure 1 *Some health hazards of development projects*

TRANSPORT

Transport systems provide a conduit for the distribution of communicable diseases such as HIV and malaria. Transport is also an important cause of traumatic injury.

 Brazil, 1970's – Half the malaria cases in Amazonia were linked to the narrow area of influence of the Transamazon Highway[11,12].

Uganda, 1986 – Along the main link road to Kenya, 32% of the truck drivers and 68% of the women working in bars were HIV positive[13].

 Papua New Guinea, 1978 – Traffic crashes and collisions were estimated to cost 1% of GNP[14].

MINING

Underground miners can suffer from permanent dust-induced lung damage and associated tuberculosis. Miners also suffer from high rates of traumatic injury.

  South Africa, 1980's – Many miners suffered from permanent dust-induced lung damage. This activates latent tuberculosis. Infection rates were 800–1,000 per 100,000[15].

 Bolivia, 1970's – The population of 24,000 mineworkers in large mines had 5,430 injuries[16].

ENERGY

The burning of both fossil fuels and biomass produces air-borne pollutants. These affect health in confined spaces and crowded cities.

 Household cooking on an open fire may be the largest single occupational health problem of women. It leads to many respiratory and eye diseases[17].

AGRICULTURE

Agricultural projects may create breeding sites for mosquitoes and other disease vectors.

 Sri Lanka, 1986 – A rice development project created breeding sites for mosquitoes which transmit Japanese encephalitis. Pigs near the rice fields provided the virus. The result was an epidemic[18].

Malnutrition is frequently a serious problem among the dependents of plantation workers and cash croppers.

Sri Lanka, 1970's – On some tea estates child labour was common, educational facilities were minimal and water facilities were inadequate. Chronic malnutrition and infant mortality rates were twice the rural average[19].

Kenya, 1980's – Most participants in dairy development projects sold the available milk for cash. They did not reserve enough milk to feed their children[20].

PUBLIC SERVICES

Coastal Asian towns constructed with inadequate drainage breed huge numbers of the mosquitoes which transmit lymphatic filariasis.

Burma, 1950's – Satellite towns built on swampy land became waterlogged during the rains. Mosquito breeding increased. Filariasis was transmitted[21].

MANUFACTURE AND TRADE

High rates of respiratory disorders, neonatal mortality and birth deformities are associated with high levels of water and air pollution. In developing countries generally, the annual rate of injuries resulting in disablement is very high.

 Cubato, Brazil, 1980's – There were 23 major industrial plants and many small operations. A high rate of respiratory disorders was associated with high levels of water and air pollution. Neonatal mortality and birth deformities increased[22,23,24].

 21–34% of injuries cause disablement in developing countries, in the UK the figure is 3%[16].

10 INITIAL SCREENING OF THE PROJECT FOR HEALTH HAZARDS

The initial screening of a project for health or other impacts is likely to be a desk exercise by a busy project officer. The officer is likely to be a specialist in the main development sector that the project addresses. This may include agriculture, engineering or economics, but rarely health. If the officer decides that there are possible health impacts then studies can be planned to describe those impacts and consider safeguards. If the officer does not consider health impacts at this stage then valuable opportunities to include health safeguards in project plans and operations will be lost.

There are two basic questions:

◆   Is the project in a health sensitive location? (*identified from maps, foci, and provincial health records*);

◆   Does the project contain health sensitive components? (*such as hazardous and hazard causing operations and materials*).

There are a number of sources of reference information that can be consulted to answer these questions.

10.1   MAPS

The World Health Organization publishes maps which indicate the distribution of various communicable diseases by country. For example, "Geographical distribution of arthropod-borne diseases and their principal vectors"[25] and "Atlas of the Global Distribution of Schistosomiasis"[26]. Figure 2 is an example.

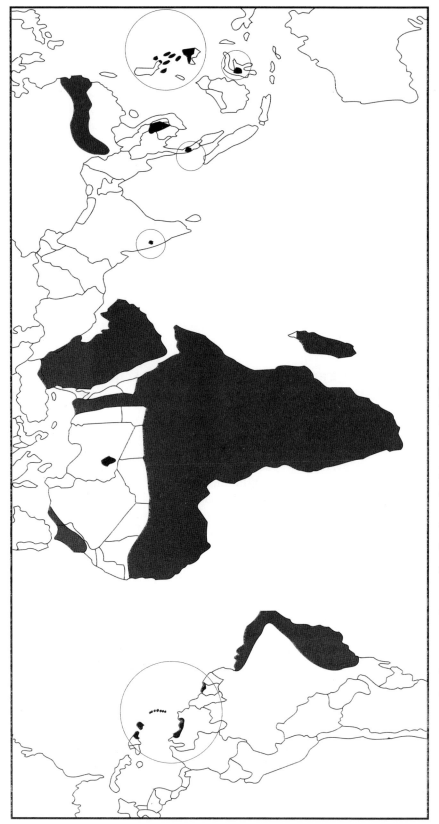

Figure 2 *Map example: the approximate distribution of schistosomiasis*[26]

Some countries publish provincial distribution maps of a range of diseases and health indicators. For example, the Department of Health, Indonesia, published maps of provincial health data in 1990[27]. The maps cover demography, malnutrition, a wide range of communicable diseases, and health service provision.

10.2 FOCI

Within each country, province or district the distribution of health hazards is patchy, or focal. It is often associated with particular topography, habitat or point sources. Figure 3 illustrates some general associations between vector-borne disease and habitat. The habitat requirements of malaria and schistosomiasis are described in more detail in later chapters.

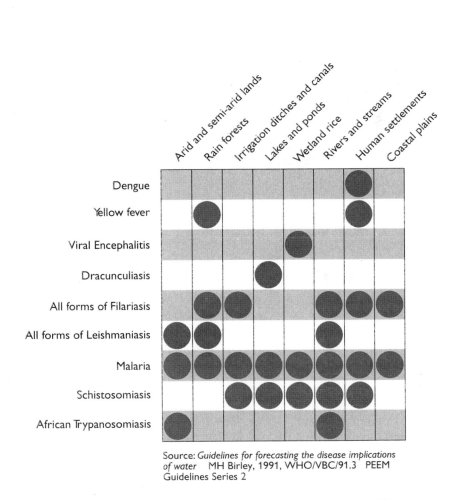

Source: *Guidelines for forecasting the disease implications of water* MH Birley, 1991, WHO/VBC/91.3 PEEM Guidelines Series 2

Figure 3 *Some associations between vector-borne disease and habitat*

10.3   NATIONAL AND PROVINCIAL HEALTH RECORDS

Many countries publish an annual list of the ten leading causes of mortality and morbidity, based on hospital records. See Table 4. The accuracy of such data is limited at both national and project level. Nevertheless, it provides an indication of existing health hazards. The health risks associated with many of these health hazards may or may not change as a result of the project.

TABLE 4   Example: The rank of ten leading causes of morbidity in the Philippines, 1988, according to hospital records.

Cause	National	Bohol District	N. Samar District
Bronchitis	1	2	1
Diarrhoeal diseases	2	1	2
Influenza	3	7	3
Pneumonias	4	3	4
Tuberculosis	5	4	5
Malaria	6		
Injuries	7	6	6
Heart Disease	8	5	9
Measles	9	8	7
Tumours	10	9	10
Inf. Hepatitis		10	
Schistosomiasis			8

10.4   AN INITIAL SCOPE FOR THE ASSESSMENT

The health hazards have been classed and described in an earlier section of this chapter (*see Types of Health Hazards, section 8*). Several health hazards may be important in each class and these may change between the construction, early and late operation stages of the project development.

The risks associated with these health hazards may depend on project location, design, operation and maintenance as well as the nature of the community. The spatial boundaries of the hazards are variable, for example reaching far downstream and downwind in some cases. It follows that the scope of the initial screening process should be very broad, so as to include all the temporal, technical, spatial and communal boundaries for the health hazards. The process successively rejects more elements and produces a tighter focus.

The following points are relevant:

◆ Health hazards which have a high frequency and severity, and which are preventable or controllable, should receive the highest priority.

◆ The most important tool for assessing what could happen is the experience of similar projects in the region.

◆ Some health hazards may not have a significant health impact until a project has been operational for more than ten years.

◆ There will always be additional hazards of importance in specific projects that were not predicted by any general review and may require contingency plans.

10.5   REVIEWS OF KNOWN HEALTH IMPACTS

The following chapters contain extensive reviews of the health hazards which have been recorded in association with specific development sectors. The review is organized by sector and establishes linkages with health hazards. The purpose of this review is to identify *potential* problems. Not all will be important in each project.

A table has been provided at the beginning of each development sector to alert the busy reader to some of the health hazards that are considered. The table also suggests the stage of the project cycle where action may be required.

11   INITIAL HEALTH EXAMINATION (IHE) OR RAPID APPRAISAL

After the project officer has flagged a concern about health impacts, an initial health examination, or rapid appraisal, is required to classify the health impacts according to Table 5. This process uses available information such

TABLE 5   Health impact classification

Classification	Interpretation
A	Significant health impacts, mitigation difficult or requires special budget
B	Significant health impacts, mitigation practical without special budget
C	No significant health impacts to local communities and affected populations

as published and unpublished reports and interviews with local specialists. It is akin to rapid rural appraisal and may involve a site visit. It may be undertaken by an officer responsible for impact assessment.

In order to make this classification it is necessary to:

◆ rank the change in health risks attributable to the project for a range of health hazards;

◆ consider possible mitigation measures;

◆ rank the possible mitigation measures by cost, practicality and acceptability.

In order to rank health risks associated with the health hazards it is necessary to construct a project profile. The profile identifies the current status of the community, their environment and their health services. It also identifies how the status will be changed by the project. The three main sub-components are:

◆ Vulnerable communities –
identify the communities who may be exposed to the health hazard and why they are vulnerable;

◆ Environmental factors –
identify the pathways by which the exposure to health hazards may occur;

◆ Capability of health protection agencies –
identify the agencies with a responsibility for safeguarding health together with their strengths and weaknesses.

The conclusions of this process can be recorded in a summary health impact assessment table. See Table 6. The table can be expanded to include a list of specific health hazards under each hazard category. The following sections describe the components in more detail. Table 8 provides an example. Chapter 13 provides a training exercise. A separate publication details the procedure for the case of vector-borne diseases and water resource development[28].

11.1   VULNERABLE COMMUNITIES

The population can be grouped according to age, sex, education, occupation, income, cultural and religious group, family size, nutritional status, behaviour, exposure or susceptibility. Groups may be difficult to identify and do not remain static. Ethnic and religious minorities, refugees, displaced populations and the very young or very old are especially vulnerable. For example, pregnant and lactating women are especially vulnerable to malaria and this is relevant to settlement siting.

Most projects are expected to be overwhelmingly beneficial to the health and economic well-being of many communities. Others, the vulnerable com-

TABLE 6   Summary Health Impact Assessment Table

Health hazard	Community vulnerability	Environmental factors	Capability of health protection agencies	Health risk attributable to project
Communicable disease				
Non-communicable disease				
Malnutrition				
Injury				
Mental disorder				

munities, may experience some adverse health consequences. Table 7 indicates the nature of some vulnerable communities.

Primary communities are those who are directly affected by the project. They will either already live in the project area or they will be immigrants. Some of them will be specifically identified as project beneficiaries.

Secondary communities are those indirectly affected by the project. For example, they may be attracted to the project site by the opportunities which it offers or displaced from land which they have traditionally used. Although these communities are not part of the project plans they may be numerically far greater than the primary communities and suffer from more severe health risks.

Many projects draw poor migrants from a wide hinterland. As they become squatters in the project area they are especially vulnerable to the diseases of poor living conditions. They retain links with their original homes and may carry diseases back with them to dependents who become vulnerable in their turn.

The needs of women in development are now widely recognized. These include specific health hazards which are changed by development projects. Amongst these are sexually transmitted diseases, including HIV infection, and domestic violence.

Community vulnerability is determined by factors such as:

◆ natural and acquired immunity to communicable disease;

◆ economic status;

◆ hazard avoidance behaviour.

TABLE 7   Examples of vulnerable communities whose health may be changed by a project

All projects

Vulnerable groups	Health hazards or exposure
Construction workers	Communicable disease, non-communicable disease, injury
Camp followers	Communicable disease, STDs
Project workforce	Communicable disease, non-communicable disease, injury
Local dependents	Malnutrition – household members are affected to different degrees
Distant dependents	Malnutrition in the labour reserve, communicable disease imported by circulating labour
Casual labour	Communicable disease
Women employees	Injury due to violence; miscarriage, fetal damage
Child labour	Communicable disease, injury
Displaced communities	Malnutrition due to loss of subsistence; stress
Resettled communities	Communicable disease, malnutrition, stress
Periphery	Non-communicable disease due to pollution; malnutrition
Downstream/downwind	Non-communicable disease due to pollution

Specific sub-sectors

Farmers and agricultural labourers	Communicable disease (including zoonoses), non-communicable disease due to agro-chemical poisoning, crop-specific hazards
Forestry workers	Communicable diseases (including malaria), injury
Tourists and tourist servers	Communicable diseases, stress related diseases
Industrial employees	Communicable disease, non-communicable disease, injury
Fishing communities	Malnutrition due to disruption of coastal resources
Migrant workers	Communicable disease, non-communicable disease, malnutrition, injury, mental disorder

Immunity is affected by factors such as prior exposure, vaccination, age and gender. Economic status affects access to health services, hazardous occupations, food security and nutrition. Techniques are available to determine these factors.

Hazard avoidance behaviour is partly determined by knowledge, attitude, belief and practice (KAP). Short surveys provide a practical tool for determining this component of community vulnerability. For example, surveys of rural communities frequently show that their knowledge of transmission of malaria is very limited. Consequently they may not attach importance to preventing mosquito bites and may take no practical action. In addition to structured surveys, informal interviews and participant observation techniques may be required.

Any survey should be preceeded by actions to encourage community participation. This will include meetings to inform communities about the project, to listen to their reaction and to agree courses of action that safeguard their interests.

CHECKLIST

◆   Have all the communities associated with the project been identified?

◆   Do any of them appear to be especially vulnerable to the project as a result of location, behaviour, exposure, age, gender or cultural reasons?

11.2   ENVIRONMENTAL FACTORS

The community is exposed to the environment through location, occupation and behaviour. The environment is changed by the project. New health hazards may be introduced and old health hazards may disappear. The changes may take place immediately or over a timescale of ten, or more, years.

Examples of hazardous environmental factors include locations, habitats and structures, such as:

◆   proximity to industrial plant;

◆   being within flight range of the breeding sites of insect vectors;

◆   a domestic water supply downstream of excreta, or industrial waste, disposal;

◆   poorly maintained irrigation ditches which serve as vector breeding sites;

◆   swamp habitats of the schistosomiasis snail host;

◆   poorly maintained roads with numerous traffic crashes and collisions.

Examples of behavioural changes that reduce exposure to a health hazard include:

◆   maintenance of irrigation ditches to prevent mosquito breeding;

◆   avoiding the swamp habitat of the schistosomiasis snail host;

◆   boiling contaminated drinking water;

◆   defensive driving.

Identification of important environmental factors is the most complex task of the IHE. For example, the environmental factors associated with vector-borne disease hazards are described in WHO's "Guidelines for Forecasting the Vector-Borne Disease Implications of Water Resources Development"[28]. These factors include: vector species, pesticide resistance, seasonality, host blood preference, breeding site requirements, reservoir hosts, flight range, and resting behaviour. Other examples are described in later chapters.

Local specialist advice should be sought from the ministry of health (divisions of environmental health, communicable disease and non-communicable disease) and the ministry of labour (occupational health and safety).

CHECKLIST

◆   Are there any features of the environment which promote exposure to health hazards?

◆   Are there any practical environmental changes that provide safeguards and mitigations?

11.3   CAPABILITY OF PROTECTION AGENCIES

In most countries, several agencies are jointly responsible for human health. The health service is responsible for routine health data collection, curative and preventative services. Environmental protection agencies regulate and monitor compliance with waste emissions, water and air quality, noise and, sometimes, occupational health and safety regulations. Ministries of man-power or labour are frequently responsible for occupational health and safety. Ministries such as public works, agriculture and industry may have EIA committees which oversee compliance with national environmental protection regulations. In many countries there are environmental legisla-tion and implementing agencies[29]. The capability of these agencies is limited by economic, staff, and infrastructure resources.

Environmental protection agencies are very new compared to health agen-cies. Their main function is regulatory. They are best at regulating pollution. They have little or no experience of regulating communicable disease, malnutrition or occupational health and safety. There are a number of programmes for strengthening their capability through technical assistance.

Health agencies have a limited regulatory function. Environmental health departments are responsible for sanitation and water and food quality inspection. These agencies have little or no experience of planning and regulating projects which are primarily associated with other sectors. They can measure the prevalence rates of communicable diseases, injuries, malnutrition and the symptoms of ill-health. Occupational health and safety may not be within their brief.

The capabilities of health agencies are surveyed by the World Health Organization. National health statistics reveal the broad differences between national capabilities. Health statistics may be inaccurate due to under-reporting. Some diseases are notifiable but compliance with notification requirements may be poor.

Very few countries are likely to have institutional procedures for minimizing vector-borne health risks through project design, although this is seminal. Many countries only have insecticide based vector control programmes, which are unsatisfactory mitigation measures.

In rural areas, access to health care may be determined by walking distance. Acceptable walking distance varies with culture, topography and poverty. An estimate of access is the percentage of the community who live within walking distance. If a road is constructed, more distant communities may gain access using public transport. It should not be assumed that accessible health care is already available.

EXAMPLES

◆ A country with an annual per capita health expenditure of under $10, such as the Philippines, may have a different capability to a country whose expenditure is over $100, such as the Cook Islands. However, some countries provide good health services at low cost. A country with an infant mortality rate of over 100/1000, such as Pakistan, has a demonstrably lower capability than Singapore, with less than 10/1000.

◆ Diarrhoeal diseases are the third principal cause of death in pre-teen Malaysians and a leading cause of paediatric hospital admissions. Incidence was greatly under-reported due to the following factors[30]:

  • Data was not reported by private practitioners.
  • Rates of under- and non-reporting were very high.
  • Terminology was not standardized (the terms gastroenteritis, diarrhoea and food poisoning were all used).
  • Specific diseases such as cholera, dysenteries and typhoid were often reported separately.

USING RATE INFORMATION

The prevalence rate is the number of cases of the condition at a particular time divided by the size of the exposed community. The rate will vary over time. It may stabilize, peak, cycle, or change with the seasons. It may be relatively stable, or unstable and epidemic. Both point of time and period of time prevalence rates are commonly used. The intensity of the condition may also vary between individuals, causing greater or lesser disability. Many diseases have a long latency period. They may not become apparent for ten or more years and cannot be easily attributed to a specific project or source of effluent.

$$Prevalence\ rate\ =\ \frac{Number\ of\ cases}{Number\ of\ people\ exposed}$$

In order to interpret data about the ill-health of a community it is crucial to use rate data. Unless the data is expressed as rates it is impossible to compare the health risk experienced by different communities or the time trend in a single community.

One simple measure of the capability of a health protection agency is the evidence that rate information is routinely being used. The skill to use rate information is far from common at both national and district level and the census data, which provides the denominator, may not be accurate. Action may be required to strengthen the capability of protection agencies through further training.

CHECKLIST

Health Services

◆ Do the project communities have realistic access to health services based on distance, cost and time to travel, opening times, drug supplies, trained personnel availability, gender and age?

◆ Are health centre diagnostic facilities functional, quality controlled, timely?

◆ Do peripheral health centres have functional water supplies and latrines as well as drug supplies and diagnostic equipment and are personnel paid regularly?

◆ Do health statistics travel down the line to the periphery as well as up to regional headquarters?

◆ Is routine health surveillance data accurate, calculated as rates, displayed in graphs, used in decision-making, of comparative or absolute value?

◆ Are the health services oriented towards monitoring and responding to new needs?

Capacity Building
◆ Do the capabilities of the environmental protection agency require strengthening?
◆ Do the capabilities of the health service require strengthening?
◆ Do the capabilities of the office responsible for occupational health and safety require strengthening?
◆ Is the ministry of health represented in the EIA procedure, project design or approval process?

12   INITIAL HEALTH EXAMINATION REPORT

The conclusions of the IHE should be presented in a brief report that accompanies the summary health impact assessment table (see Table 6).

The report should indicate the project type and location. These were used in the initial screening to identify health hazards. The health hazards are grouped by their main categories. There are many different hazards in each category. The health risk depends on the community exposure to the hazard, the environmental factors which promote that exposure and the capability of protection agencies, such as the health service, to safeguard health. Simple scores should be used such as: unchanged, increasing, decreasing, low, high.

As there may be health risks even if the project is not implemented, only the change in health risk is strictly associated with the project.

The following example illustrates how an Initial Health Examination was completed for an irrigation project in the Philippines (see Table 8).

12.1   AN EXAMPLE FROM THE PHILIPPINES

MALARIA

Malaria is variably endemic throughout the Philippines with an epidemic potential and multiple drug resistance. Vector breeding is restricted to shaded streams and irrigation ditches. Successful watershed reforestation may create a vector habitat in about ten years. Good maintenance of watersheds and irrigation ditches would minimize the risk. If the surveillance system remains locally operational it should be able to respond to renewed transmission.

SCHISTOSOMIASIS

Schistosomiasis is endemic at and near the project site. The snail vector inhabits streams and rice fields. Proper operation and maintenance would minimize this risk. There is an active surveillance system and curative drugs are available but there is a local staff shortage.

TABLE 8   Example of a Summary Initial Health Examination

Project Title: Small Water Impoundment Multipurpose (SWIM) Project
Project type: Multipurpose irrigation, with watershed management
Location: Visayas, Philippines
Date of assessment: April, 1991
Community group: Farmers and farm labourers

Health hazard	Community vulnerability	Environmental factors	Health service capability	Health risk (associated with project)
Malaria	Susceptibility is high and labour migration may introduce the parasite	Vector habitat depends on reforestation	Curative – drug resistance Surveillance – localized Vector control – in response to outbreaks	Variable. Check in ten years after significant reforestation
Schistosomiasis	Leading cause of local morbidity, severe cases reported	Snail populations surveyed at project site	Curative, snail control and surveillance, but staff shortage	High risk, but mitigation practical
Dengue Haemorrhagic Fever	Low in rural areas	Vector widespread	Hospitalization of cases	Very low and unchanged
Encephalitis (J.E.)	Low, no cases reported	Vectors probable	Supportive treatment	Very low and unchanged
Pesticide poisoning	High – poor education	Increasing agricultural usage of extremely toxic substances	Vigilance probably low	Moderate, increasing, mitigation required
Malnutrition	High but reducing with improved income	Intensive rice production, fisheries	High	Moderate, check that fish consumption increases as planned
Injury	Low	Draught animal power	Casualty ward	Low, unchanged
Enteric and other helminth infections	High prevalence	Tube wells, open defecation, no domestic water supply component	Curative	Unchanged, but domestic water supply required

DENGUE

Dengue is largely restricted to towns and cities where population density is high.

JAPANESE ENCEPHALITIS

Japanese encephalitis is rare in the Philippines. The vector probably occurs locally but there is probably no reservoir of infection. Pigs can be an important reservoir host but no intensive pig rearing is planned at the project site.

PESTICIDE POISONING

Pesticide poisoning has been recognized as an important health hazard of intensive rice cultivation in the Philippines. Farmers are poorly informed of appropriate methods of handling pesticides. Agricultural promotion emphasizes pest resistant varieties of rice and integrated pest management (IPM) methods, but this may not be adopted by local farmers. Little pesticide is currently being used at the project sites but an increase is foreseen. Extremely hazardous pesticides are on sale locally and continuing efforts are required to restrict their use.

MALNUTRITION

Malnutrition is a recognized problem. Improvement is expected in the income of farmers and farm labourers without reduction of subsistence crops. Proposed fish aquaculture may improve the diet, if implemented.

INJURY

Injury associated with farm machinery is unlikely to become a problem as draught animals are commonly used.

ENTERIC INFECTION

Enteric infections associated with diarrhoea and typhoid are among the leading causes of morbidity. Geohelminth infection is common. The drinking water supply is drawn from open wells and open defecation is common. The programme contains no components which will reduce this health risk. Safe domestic water supply is required.

RATING

The project is rated B with the recommendation that action is taken to strengthen local health education through agricultural extension so as to prevent schistosomiasis and pesticide poisoning. The community should be consulted regarding domestic water supply.

13   MITIGATION MEASURES

In order to complete the project classification it is necessary to consider the available mitigation measures. These are discussed in more detail under Risk Management below. A complete discussion lies outside the range of this book.

Possible mitigation measures could be grouped into the following classes:

◆   Opportunities for modifying project location.

◆   Opportunities for modifying project design.

◆   Opportunities for modifying project operation and maintenance.

◆   Opportunities for incorporating environmental management measures.

◆   Opportunities for strengthening health services.

◆   Need for monitoring and surveillance (*how will the data be used?*).

Each mitigation measure on the list should be roughly classified in terms of:

◆   Affordability (*is it cheap to build?*).

◆   Sustainability (*is it cheap to maintain? is it easy to operate?*).

◆   Acceptability (*is it socially acceptable to the local community?*).

◆   Accessibility (*is it physically, socially or economically accessible to the vulnerable communities?*).

◆   Cost-effectiveness (*could the resources needed for this mitigation measure be more effectively employed elsewhere?*).

14   HEALTH IMPACT ASSESSMENT

14.1   WHICH PROJECTS REQUIRE A FULL HEALTH IMPACT ASSESSMENT?

At this stage the project can be classed into the categories listed in Table 5. The project may also receive a classification from environmental and social assessments.

The project officer must then decide whether a full health impact assessment, requiring the services of a specialist consultant, is necessary. The decision will depend on the available experience and expertise within the responsible agency.

If an HIA is required, a terms of reference, TOR, will be prepared for a specialist consultant. The Initial Health Examination will have identified the health hazards and communities which the TOR should address. The health risk assessment will seek to establish in more detail whether changes in the principal health risks can be attributed to the project. Mitigation measures will also be considered in more detail.

14.2   COMPONENTS OF HIA

As a result of the Initial Health Examination, the HIA can focus, in depth, on a small number of significant health hazards. During the feasibility study, the consultant should assess the health risk associated with each health hazard at each project stage and for each vulnerable community. The assessment is concerned with the change in exposure associated with the project: identifying the communities which will be exposed and the nature, magnitude and likelihood of that exposure. The consultant should also establish the capabilities of existing protection agencies, including the health service, to monitor, inform, safeguard and mitigate health risk. The description of the existing conditions is often referred to as profiling.

The conclusions of the assessment must be presented to the decision makers in a format which will enable them to use the information effectively. The same summary table used for Initial Health Examination is recommended.

The cycle of hazard identification and risk interpretation may have to be repeated. First, as a rapid appraisal and second as a detailed study of the major risks. The feasibility study should provide the information required for negotiating changes in project plans or operation to safeguard health.

14.3   SCOPING

During preparation of the TOR it will be necessary to establish the boundaries for the consultant. These will include the hazards to be addressed, the communities of interest, the spatial boundaries and temporal stages for which a prediction is required. One of the consultant's tasks will be to refine the scope.

Discussions may be held with other agencies concerned with the project. Public meetings may be organised. Community participation should be actively sought out.

THE SPATIAL BOUNDARY

The influence of a project extends far beyond the project site. The economic opportunities draw formal and informal labour which retain links with distant communities. Vectors breeding on site disperse downwind. Effluent discharged into streams and air flows are carried many kilometres. Toxins may accumulate in the food-chain and affect the health of communities to whom the food is exported.

EXAMPLES

◆ In chemical plants, the scope may include the whole of the flow-cycle from extraction of raw materials through to waste disposal, the lifetime of the workforce and the spatial limits at which gaseous discharges can be detected.

◆ Schistosomiasis in Ethiopia was distributed between river basins by seasonal labourers who worked on an irrigation scheme[31].

◆ Malaria mosquitoes usually fly less than about 2km in search of a blood-meal. They can migrate much greater distances when assisted by the wind[32].

◆ A large project was completed to supply a city with a new piped sewerage system. The engineering focus was on removing raw sewage from the city streets. The main sewerage pipes led to a primary treatment plant. The septic fluid was then discharged into open drains which were beyond the bounds of the engineering project. The unfenced drains flowed through densely populated suburbs and the community had intimate contact with the septic fluid, even extracting it for domestic use. The boundary of the health impact assessment had to be larger than the boundary of the engineering problem.

THE TEMPORAL BOUNDARY

Four main project stages may be identified:

◆ pre-project;

◆ construction;

◆ early operation;

◆ late operation (after 10 years).

In many cases, the health hazards are present and causing substantial health risks independently of the project. A prediction is required of the change in project related risks during the lifetime of the project.

Some health risks may become apparent immediately. Others may remain unapparent until the late project stage. Risks which have long latency periods may not normally be considered in development planning. However, they may be seminal to health impact assessment. See Table 3 for examples.

14.4 GENERIC TERMS OF REFERENCE FOR HEALTH IMPACT ASSESSMENT

A Generic Terms of Reference for Health Impact Assessment could include the following components:

INTRODUCTION

This states the purpose of the terms of reference, the type of project to be assessed, and the implementing arrangements for the health impact assessment.

BACKGROUND INFORMATION

This provides a brief project description with the objectives, the status and timetable, and the project proponent. Related projects within the region must be identified.

OBJECTIVES

This states the general as well as specific objectives of the health impact assessment in relation to the project preparatory activities such as feasibility studies (planning, design and execution) and as part of environmental impact assessment.

ENVIRONMENTAL REQUIREMENTS

This section identifies regulations and guidelines which will govern the assessment such as operational directives, national laws or regulations, regional or provincial regulations, and specific regulations of other funding organizations involved in the project. The requirement for health impact studies may be included in the EIA regulations.

STUDY AREA

This specifies the boundaries of the study area for the assessment. It should include the human communities downstream and downwind of the project. The HIA boundaries could go beyond the EIA boundaries, which are usually the watershed or airshed.

SCOPE OF WORK

The health hazards and communities that require particular attention are obtained from the Initial Health Examination Summary Table. The consultant could be asked to refine the scope of work for contracting agency review and approval. Other agencies may be invited to comment and public meetings may be held.

HEALTH RISK ASSESSMENT

The consultant will assess the health risk associated with each health hazard at each project stage. The assessment will include the following considerations:

COMMUNITY VULNERABILITY

Identify each vulnerable community to be affected by the project and assess the nature, magnitude and likelihood of exposure. Estimate the prevalence rate of each hazard in each vulnerable community from health sector records and/or special survey.

ENVIRONMENTAL FACTORS

Consider the environmental factors that may contribute to an increase in health risk and define mitigating measures as input to project planning. Estimate the magnitude of the factors.

CAPABILITY OF PROTECTION AGENCIES

Establish in more detail the capabilities of existing protection agencies, such as the environmental and health agencies, which have jurisdiction over the project site. The consultant should assess the limitations of existing data and recommend how to strengthen health information systems to meet requirements for health risk management.

HEALTH RISK MANAGEMENT

The consultant may be asked to formulate a monitoring programme during the construction and operational stages which includes: a description of the work tasks, skills/tests/interviews, frequency, institutional and financial arrangements, justification/use of the monitoring data. The consultant should define the safeguards and mitigating measures required as inputs to the feasibility study.

CONTEXT FOR HEALTH RISK MANAGEMENT

Account should be taken of the availability of resources and funds, whether there are any interest groups actively concerned about the project and its health impact, whether local environmental lobby groups exist, the attitudes of local authorities and government, and whether meetings have been held to promote changes in the project. Consideration should be given to any groups which may oppose change, and any groups whose support could be obtained in order to increase the prospect of protective/mitigating measures being applied.

CONSULTANT REQUIREMENTS

Ideally, the consultant would have previous experience of assessing the health impacts of development projects. However, the consultant must have specialist knowledge of the most significant health risks identified during the Initial Health Examination. If diverse health risks were identified then additional consultants may be required with specialist knowledge of each.

REPORTS, DURATION AND SCHEDULE

This will specify the total period of the study, staff-months of experts, dates for consultation, periodic reports and other target dates.

OTHER INFORMATION

This will provide the consultant(s) with preliminary information on data sources, background reports and studies, and other relevant publications.

14.5   HEALTH IMPACT STATEMENT

The output from an HIA will be a health impact statement. This should be modelled on the Initial Health Examination. It should include a summary table similar to Table 6. The table should be supported by an explanation of each item.

15   HEALTH RISK MANAGEMENT

The risk assessment is presented to a project approval committee who must evaluate the relative importance of the impacts which have been identified in a wider context. They will decide the priority to attach to the recommended safeguards and mitigation measures, negotiate resources and assign monitoring and surveillance tasks.

Risk management consists of incorporating safeguards and mitigation measures in project design and operation. Safeguarding entails proposing modifications to project plans and operations and ensuring that the capability exists for effective mitigation. This could include strengthening of protection agency capabilities.

Mitigation entails vigilant monitoring for the lifetime of the project accompanied by appropriate and timely response to increasing health risks. Monitoring depends on an adequate health information system. Response may depend, for example, on stocks of insecticides and drugs and their dissemination and use.

In industrial projects a hierarchy of risk management measures has been defined which may be of general utility. These are:

◆ Elimination of the source of hazard;

◆ Substitution of hazardous processes and materials by those which are less hazardous;

◆ Geographical or physical isolation of hazards from vulnerable communities, for example by land zonation;

◆ Use of engineering controls to reduce the health risk. For example, build structures with stronger walls in order to avoid catastrophic failures;

◆ Adoption of safe working practices, such as regular equipment maintenance;

◆ Use of personal protective equipment, such as rubber gloves or bednets.

Table 9 indicates some of the actions and concerns which should be addressed during each project stage. A similar table is included at the beginning of each development sector. The objective is to alert the development planner to issues that should be addressed at each project stage.

Where the community is exposed to a hazard as a result of occupation, mitigation may be achieved primarily by occupational safety measures and continuous health education. Where the community is exposed through its location, mitigation may be achieved primarily by reducing the hazard or relocation. At the planning stage land-use zonation and resettlement siting could be considered. Table 10 lists examples of suitable interventions for controlling health hazards of the work environment.

TABLE 9 Health risk management: some possible actions at different project stages

Project stage	Surveillance and monitoring	Health service provision	Safety provision and preventive measures	Obtaining advice from the health sector about:
Location	Site specific health hazards, general health status of local communities, ten most common causes of morbidity and mortality, location and functioning of health services	Access to health services	Settlement siting	Disease foci, vector biology
Planning and design	Improve routine health service surveillance by: retraining, health information system, laboratory services	Health centre, trained personnel, drug supply, equipment maintenance, housing for health workers, casualty/emergency unit	OHS planning, traffic routing, environmental management	Communicable disease control, environmental management for vector control, environmental manipulation, environmental health
Construction	OHS monitoring, environmental health: water supply, sanitary system, drug supply, vector monitoring	STD clinic, distribution of condoms, health training, casualty/emergency unit, vector and other communicable disease control	Safety measures consistent with local economy, OHS training, traffic routing	Communicable disease control, environmental health
Operation	Routine medical examination, action oriented disease trend analysis, child growth monitoring, OHS monitoring, infant mortality monitoring, vector monitoring, casualty rates	Health education, immunization, obstetrics, training traditional health workers, food supplement programme, casualty/emergency unit, access to health service outside working hours, vector and other communicable disease control	OHS implementation, environmental management	Communicable disease control, environmental management for vector control, environmental manipulation, environmental health, human behaviour modification
Opportunities for project enhancement	Health information system, diagnostic/laboratory services	Healthy workforce is more productive and vice versa	Safer working methods, training, injury compensation	Intersectoral collaboration

TABLE 10   Controlling hazards in the work environment.

Intervention	Example
Substitution	Replacing asbestos with cement materials.
Dust suppression	Wetting products to avoid them becoming airborne and posing a respiratory hazard.
Enclosure	Conducting shot-blasting in an enclosed booth or a separate area.
Segregation	Separating non-dusty operations (eg. quality control) from those generating dust. Doing maintenance work out of normal production hours thus decreasing exposure to dust.
Exhaust ventilation	Removal of dust and chemicals from processes.
General ventilation	Improving airflow through plant generally while making sure that fresh air rather than dusty air circulates more.
Personal protective equipment	Respirators for those exposed to dust which cannot otherwise be controlled: these have to be of the appropriate standard and need to be maintained; ear protectors; boots; gloves; helmets.
Labelling of hazardous materials	Making it clear that certain materials are likely to be poisonous or otherwise hazardous; informing workers of the meaning of such labels.
Good housekeeping	Keeping plants generally tidy, not leaving chemicals lying around.
Education, information and training	Involving all personnel and trades union representatives in learning about health hazards and developing appropriate measures to control dust and other adverse exposures.
Inspection and monitoring	Of dust levels, engineering controls and general factory conditions.

Environmental management for vector control is an example of a mitigation where project design is seminal.

15.1 ENVIRONMENTAL MANAGEMENT

Agricultural development and infrastructure projects, in particular, provide an opportunity for vector-borne disease control through environmental management. Environmental management for vector control consists of deliberate alteration of the environment, environmental factors or interactions between people and the environment designed to limit vector breeding, survival or human contact. The environment includes soil, water, vegetation and urban and rural settlements. The environmental factors include microclimate, chemical composition and vector behaviour.

Environmental Management for Vector Control can be summarized as follows:

◆　Permanent modification to the environment to inhibit vector breeding.

◆　Repetitive actions, such as weed removal, to inhibit vector breeding.

◆　Changes in human behaviour and habitation which reduce breeding or exposure.

◆　Timely assessment of the health hazards to ensure that design changes can be incorporated in project plans and operations.

Some elements of the first three are discussed in WHO's "Manual on Environmental Management for Mosquito Control"[33]. They include the following measures:

◆　Drainage of urban and rural settlements and irrigation systems.

◆　Alteration of river, reservoir and other water impoundment levels by sluicing and flushing.

◆　Alteration of water salinity.

◆　Removal of favourable and planting of unfavourable vegetation for vector breeding.

◆　Changing conditions of exposure to sunlight and shade.

◆　Land filling and levelling.

◆　Alternate flooding and drying of rice fields.

◆　Destruction of water-filled containers; screening of cisterns.

◆　Improvements in sanitation, sewerage and solid waste management systems.

◆　Siting human settlements 2km or more from vector sources.

◆　Land zonation.

◆　Using livestock as diversionary hosts.

◆　Using bednets and house screens.

◆　Management of irrigation water.

◆　Avoidance of infested water for domestic use or recreation.

Many of these measures cannot easily be incorporated in project design or operation unless previously identified through health impact assessment. Environmental management requires collaboration at all levels between different public sectors, the pooling of expertise and the involvement of the community.

EXAMPLES

◆ Resettlement sites could be located at least 2km from vector breeding sites, such as the forest margin. Irrigation ditches could be self-draining when not in use. A proportion of water taxes could be retained under local control and used for project maintenance. Foot-bridges could be provided where schistosomiasis vectors are present. Rice cultivation could be intensive and synchronous to inhibit vectors. Water storage jars could be fitted with tight lids. Intermittent piped water supply could be avoided. Solid waste could be prevented from collecting rainwater or blocking drains. Septic tanks could be properly sealed. Downstream sections of dammed rivers could be regularly flushed.

15.2   STANDARDS FOR AIR, WATER AND NOISE

The emissions from new and existing industrial projects are hazardous to health and the risk is dose related. National and international standards have been determined for many emissions. There are many sources of error that complicate the problem of defining appropriate thresholds. The standards are usually set following studies on experimental animals supported by epidemiology. Critical doses are determined at which the majority of the most vulnerable community are considered safe. Risk management is then a matter of ensuring that emission standards are designed into new plant and conscientiously followed. Unfortunately, unscrupulous managers may seek to circumvent the regulations by, for example, increasing the emissions during the night. Affordable systems of monitoring are required to police emissions. In cases where the emission is easily detected by its colour, smell, taste or sound and is not immediately hazardous to health, the local community may be an effective and economical source of monitoring information.

15.3   MONITORING AND SURVEILLANCE

Surveillance is sometimes defined as systematic measurement of variables and processes for the purpose of establishing a time trend. Monitoring, by contrast, is collecting data for analysis and action.

There is a need for health and safety monitoring in development projects, especially in cases where the health risk cannot safely be forecast. However, it is not always clear what minimum health indicators should be measured. The health service does not usually have the resources to undertake surveillance. There are problems of enforcement and there may be no institutional mechanisms able to react to changing health risks at the project level.

There is frequently a seasonal pattern to morbidity and mortality.

A distinction may be drawn between the monitoring of hazardous factors in the environment and the monitoring of human health. The link between the two is the degree of human exposure.

Environmental health monitoring systems are available to monitor water quality, hazardous discharges in air, water and solid waste, and food safety. Entomological services, based in communicable disease control departments of the health ministry, monitor the distribution and abundance of disease vectors.

The monitoring/surveillance of human health is the role of epidemiology. WHO's "Manual of Epidemiology for District Health Management" is of considerable assistance to the non-health specialist[34].

Routine government health sector surveillance data is unlikely to be sufficiently accurate, sensitive or to have the coverage needed to indicate changes in health risk associated with a specific development project. Further, the linkage between the project and community health may be so indirect that health change cannot be attributed to the project. It may be necessary to commission special surveys.

There may be a need for proxy (or surrogate) health indicators. A sewerage project might measure the number of sewage spillages. A drainage project might monitor the biting density of the common mosquito, *Culex quinquefasciatus*, as an indicator of both drainage obstruction and filariasis transmission potential.

For non-communicable disease, it may be easier to monitor the concentration of a contaminant than to monitor changes in human health. Further, health risk management requires control of the contaminant at source. The health changes associated with the contaminant may be acute or chronic. Long latency periods are possible. In either case, health monitoring is beset by problems of ethics, random error, diagnostic limitations, non-linear dose-response curves, and synergistic effects of other contaminants.

15.4 LIMITATIONS OF HEALTH SECTOR DATA

The accuracy, timeliness and coverage of national health data in developing countries are variable. Population statistics, the denominator in many rate calculations, may often be 6–15 years out of date as national censuses are infrequent and may take years to analyze. Such data is frequently inaccurate when applied to small areas. Births and deaths are frequently under-reported by as much as 50%. The cause of death is also poorly classified.

Hospital morbidity statistics are also poor. They may be based on unconfirmed diagnoses or inadequate knowledge of the size of population served.

Environmental health data include pollution monitoring, occupational injuries and food safety. They are collected by many agencies other than the health sector. The quality is sometimes excellent but access is limited by considerations of sensitivity and confidentiality. General conclusions cannot be extrapolated to local areas.

Data collection systems have often been designed for surveillance rather than monitoring. Consequently, the data are not used for management and are inappropriate, under-valued and poorly stored.

15.5   HEALTH SERVICE PREPAREDNESS

The project planners should inform the health sector of the project plan. If a large influx of formal or informal settlers is expected then the health sector will require time to construct additional health centres, train personnel, obtain drug supplies and negotiate an increased budget. There is often an implicit assumption that the health service has the prior capacity, within its existing resources, to cope with any effects that may occur. This is unrealistic.

16   REFERENCES

1 World Health Organization Commission on Health and Environment, "Our Planet, Our Health." (World Health Organization, Geneva 1992).
2 G Gunatilleke Ed., "Health Dimensions of Economic Reform." (World Health Organization, Geneva 1992).
3 D E C Cooper Weil, A P Alicbusan, J F Wilson, M R Reich, and D J Bradley, "The Impact of Development Policies on Health: A Review of the Literature." (World Health Organization, Geneva 1990).
4 Asian Development Bank, "Guidelines for the Health Impact of Development Projects." *ADB Environment Papers*, No 11, Ed. *Office of the Environment Asian Development Bank*, (Asian Development Bank, Office of the Environment, Manila 1992).
5 M Tiffen, "Guidelines for the Incorporation of Health Safeguards into Irrigation Projects Through Intersectoral Cooperation." *PEEM Guidelines, No.1*, (WHO/FAO/UNEP, 1989).
6 V T Covello, J L Mumpower, P J M Stallen, and V R R Uppuluri Ed., "Environmental Impact Assessment, Technology Assessment, and Risk Analysis." *Series G: Ecological Sciences Vol 4.* vol. 4 (Springer-Verlag, Berlin 1985).
7 K R Smith, "Managing the risk transition." *Toxicology and Industrial Health.* 1991, 7:5/6:319–327.

8   T Harpham, "Urbanization and mental disorder." in-*The Principles of Social Psychiatry, Ed. D Bhugra and J Leff.* (Blackwell, Oxford 1993).

9   World Commission on Environment and Development, "Our Common Future." (Oxford University Press, Oxford 1987).

10 World Bank, "World Development Report 1993." (Oxford University Press, New York 1993).

11 S K Ault, "Effect of demographic patterns, social structure, and human behaviour on malaria." in-*Demography and Vector-Borne Diseases, Ed. M W Service.* (CRC Press, Florida 1989).

12 C E A Coimbra, "Human factors in the epidemiology of malaria in the Brazilian Amazon." *Hum Org.* 1988, 47:3:254–260.

13 J W Carswell, "HIV infections in healthy persons in Uganda." *AIDS.* 1987, 1:223–227.

14 J D J Havard, "World Health Organization Assignment Report." (1978) World Health Organization Regional Office for the Western Pacific. ICP/HSD/015.

15 R M Packard, "Industrial production, health and disease in sub-Saharan Africa." *Soc Sci Med.* 1989, 28:5:475–496.

16 M A El-Batawi, "Special problems of occupational health in the developing countries." in-*Occupational Health Practice, Ed. R S F Schilling.* 2nd ed., (Butterworths, London 1981).

17 World Health Organization Commission on Health and Environment, "Report of the Panel on Energy." (World Health Organization, Geneva 1992).

18 International Rice Research Institute, "Vector-borne Disease Control in Humans Through Rice Agroecosystem Management." (International Rice Research Institute, Manila 1988).

19 R Laing, "Health and Health Services for Plantation Workers: Four Case Studies." *EPC Publication No.10,* (Evaluation and Planning Centre for Health Care, London School of Hygiene and Tropical Medicine, London 1986).

20 A A J Jansen, H T Horelli, and V J Quinn, "Food and Nutrition in Kenya: A Historical Review." (University of Nairobi and UNICEF, Nairobi 1987).

21 W W Macdonald, "Control of *Culex quinquefasciatus* in Myanmar (Burma) and India: 1960–1990." *Ann Trop Med Parasit.* 1991, 85:165–172.

22 R W Findley, "Pollution control in Brazil." *Ecol Law Qtrly.* 1988, 15:1:1–68.

23 J C P Pimenta, "Multinational corporations and industrial pollution in Sao Paulo, Brazil." in-*Multinational Corporations, Environment and the Third World, Ed. C S Pearson.* (Duke University Press, Durham 1987).

24 V Thomas, "Pollution Control in Sao Paulo, Brazil: Costs, Benefits and Effects on Industrial Location." (November 1981) The World Bank. Staff Working Paper No.501.

25 World Health Organization, "Geographical Distribution of Arthropod-borne Diseases and their Principal Vectors." (WHO, Geneva 1989).

26 J P Doumenge, K E Mott, C Cheung, D Villenave, O Chapuis, M F Perrin, and G Reaud-Thomas, "Atlas of the Global Distibution of Schistosomiasis." (World Health Organization, Geneva 1987).

27 Department of Health Republic of Indonesia, "Health Problem Map by Province, Indonesia." (Department of Health, Republic of Indonesia, Jakarta 1990).

28 M H Birley, "Guidelines for Forecasting the Vector-Borne Disease Implications of Water Resources Development." *PEEM Guidelines, No. 2, Ed. PEEM Secretariat,* 2nd ed., WHO/CWS/91.3 (World Health Organization, Geneva 1991).

29 Asian Development Bank, "Environmental Legislation and Administration: Briefing Profiles of Selected Developing Member Countries of the Asian Development Bank." *ADB Environment Papers, No 2, Ed. Environment Division Asian Development Bank*, (ADB, Manila 1988).

30 S Lonergan, and T Vansickle, "Relationship between water quality and human health: a case study of the Linggi river basin in Malaysia." *Soc Sci Med*. 1991, 33:8:937–946.

31 H Kloos, "Water resource development and schistosomiasis ecology in the Awash Valley, Ethiopia." *Soc Sci Med*. 1985, 20:6:609–625.

32 M H Birley, Personal observation.

33 World Health Organization, "Manual on Environmental Management for Mosquito Control – With Special Emphasis on Malaria Vectors." (WHO, Geneva 1982).

34 J P Vaughan, and R H Morrow Ed., "Manual of Epidemiology for District Health Management." (WHO, Geneva 1989).

chapter 2

There are several issues that occur as a component of so many different development activities that they require separate attention. Of particular concern are projects which cause or contribute to population growth and population movement. Development projects may change fertility and hence the size of the vulnerable population of pregnant women and infants. The relationship is complex and outside the scope of this review.

Disruption of the social environment provides a high risk situation for transmission of diseases such as HIV. Individuals may experience feelings of powerlessness, and lack of control over their lives, separation from partners, reduced social concern about casual sexual relationships, worry about immediate provision of food, use of alcohol and other addictive drugs as well as a lack of information and resources. This may be exacerbated by homelessness, landlessness, unemployment, rapid periurban settlement, migration, population relocation and poverty[1].

1 LABOUR MOBILITY

Mobile populations are vulnerable to new health hazards. They include temporary labourers and resettlers. The accompanying table illustrates a more complete typography with examples of associated activities and health hazards[2]. Many different kinds of population movement may occur in response to a development project.

Economic development of plantations, mines and other industries have usually been accompanied by labour mobility. Temporary workers, drawn from a largely underdeveloped hinterland, are exposed to severe health hazards. These hazards are generally occupational, such as the exposure to dusts and toxic chemicals, or associated with poor living conditions. Tuberculosis, pneumoconioses and pneumonia are common[3]. Migrant workers are also vulnerable to psychiatric disorders[4,5,6,7].

EXAMPLE

◆ More than 3,000 construction workers are involved in building the Narmada Dam and associated irrigation structure in India. They are from other areas and live without their families[8].

TABLE 1   Economic activities, population mobility and examples of association with health hazards (After Prothero and Gould[2]).

	Circulation				Migration	
	Daily	**Periodic**	**Seasonal**	**Long-term**	**Irregular**	**Regular**
Rural–Rural	Cultivating (1)	Hunting (1)	Pastoralism (1,2)	Labouring (1,2)	Nomadism (1,2)	Resettlement (1,3)
Rural–Urban	Commuting (1)	Trading (1,2,3)	Labouring (1)	Labouring (1,2,3)	Drought (1,2,3)	Labouring (1,2,3)
Urban–Rural	Cultivating (1)	Trading (1)	Labouring (1)	Trading (1,2)	Refugees (1,2,3)	Retirement (1)
Urban–Urban	Commuting (1)	Trading (1,3)	Trading (1)	Relocation (3)	Refugees (3)	(3)

Health hazards
(1) Communicable disease (eg: vector-borne diseases, STDs, measles, poliomyelitis).
(2) Malnutrition/Injury.
(3) Mental disorder (eg: problems of adjustment, alcoholism).

Increasingly, women are forming part of the migrating work force as rural demand for their labour decreases. They migrate to new industrial developments in the cities or to concentrations of male labour.

Migrant labourers may choose to remain when a construction project is completed. They may create new settlements without infrastructure, live in unsanitary conditions and contribute to disputes over land and common property resources[10].

EXAMPLES

◆ Female headed households are more likely to live in poverty, in substandard housing with unsafe drinking water and inadequate sewers and with insufficient income to eat a balanced diet[9].

◆ Thirty per cent. of the temporary population of 4000 associated with the construction of the Kamburu dam in Kenya chose to remain there[10].

1.1 COMMUNICABLE DISEASE

Migrant labour systems worldwide present high risk situations for communicable disease transmission, such as HIV. Many labourers are single males who are separated from their families and communities. STD transmission is commonplace. Workers' accommodation is often intolerable, insecure and depressing[11]. The high price, legislation and poor quality of urban dwellings forces migrant workers to live apart from their families. These men seek companionship with women living near their place of work, posing a high risk for multipartner sexual activity and the spread of sexually transmitted diseases including HIV infection. One major cause of heterosexual spread of HIV in Africa has been ascribed to the special prominence of labour mobility in that region[11].

EXAMPLES

- The prevalence of STDs often increases during the harvesting season[12].

- In Nairobi, 94% of those infected with STDs were working more than 400 km from their native area[13].

- In Kampala, half of STD patients came from the surrounding rural area and half were migrants[14].

Wage employment for women is often harder to obtain or poorer paid than for men[9]. Women in such a position are at risk from sexual harassment and rape and some, perhaps many, become sex workers. Others may be required to exchange sexual favours for food and accommodation. Boys and young men may do the same. There is evidence that heterosexual STD transmission was restricted in South African mine workers by homosexual practices[15,16].

EXAMPLE

- Impoverishment, rapid urbanisation, anonymity of city life, migrant labour, poor wages and dependency of women were identified as the main factors leading to women seeking sex in exchange for money in Bulawayo, Zimbabwe[17].

Returning labourers may carry new communicable diseases to their place of origin, where health care facilities are frequently poor[18]. These include STDs that lead to female infertility[19]. Migrant workers and militia may have been the means by which a cholera epidemic moved from Tanzania to most of Southern Africa between 1978 and 1983[20].

EXAMPLES

◆ A study showed that 60% of miners diagnosed as having tuberculosis while working in South Africa died within 2 years of returning home[18].

◆ A study of daily agricultural workers in Jimma, Ethiopia, showed a higher prevalence of tuberculosis and pneumonia as compared to the general population[3].

It has been predicted that the next epidemic of HIV will be in populations of migrant workers, in rapidly urbanising populations, and among the indigenous populations of the world much affected by STDs and alcohol use[1].

1.2   NON-COMMUNICABLE DISEASE

Returning labourers may have occupational diseases for which industry has failed to accept responsibility. The burden for their care falls on their families. Some conditions, such as asbestosis, or malignant mesothelioma, a cancer of the lining of the lung due to asbestos exposure, may be especially disabling.

1.3   MALNUTRITION

The hinterland itself may be a dependent labour reserve with declining agriculture, labour shortage, poor health care facilities and malnutrition. The burden of both agricultural production and care of dependents falls more heavily on the women who are left behind. Crop production may then shift to more easily grown but less nutritious staples; child care may decline. Malnutrition and disease susceptibility may increase. The family may not be able to leave the impoverished land without losing their claim to it[19]. On the other hand, remittances from migrants may raise household incomes and provide access to a wider range of food.

EXAMPLE

◆ A study of a rural labour reserve, the Bemba, in Zambia during the 1930's concluded that labour shortage prevented bush clearing, leading to overuse of cultivated areas and a shift to less nutritious crops such as cassava[21].

---

2   RESETTLEMENT

Two important forms of resettlement are: settlement of new lands to achieve a public good; displacement to resettlement as part of the attainment of a public good. In the former case the settled community represents a productive resource and will receive support. In the latter case the community are viewed as an obstacle to development that may receive either negligible or inappropriate support[22,23]. Health hazards are rarely seen as a major constraint to resettlement success compared with problems of administration or agricultural planning.

EXAMPLES

◆ 56,000 Tonga people were displaced to resettlement by the Kariba Dam. A subsequent study noted that: disruption of social routines lasted more than five years; the community became hostile to government; local leaders lost their legitimacy; and the community were less willing to accept innovations in health care[23].

◆ The social structure of indigenous people displaced by the Ok Tedi mine in Papua New Guinea has been disrupted. Alcohol abuse has become common and women's status has been lowered[24].

Resettlement projects are also planned as a response to spontaneous population migrations, perhaps as a result of civil disturbance. In this case new infrastructure may accelerate spontaneous migration into the area.

2.1   COMMUNICABLE DISEASE

Vector-borne communicable diseases are often significant in resettlement schemes because of increased exposure or the creation of new vector-breeding sites. Careful planning and siting can do much to mitigate this risk.

EXAMPLE

◆ Resettled communities in Southeast Asia have established sub-sistence farm plots within the forest reserve. The prevalence of malaria has increased as it is largely confined to the forest and forest fringe[25].

2.2   MALNUTRITION

Communities displaced to resettlement face formidable obstacles with profound health consequences. Often no compensation has been provided. In other cases, compensation has consisted of agricultural development. This usually involves a shift from subsistence to cash cropping that the community may not accept. *See also Agriculture, chapter 6.*

EXAMPLES

◆ There may eventually be 300,000 resettlers from the Narmada project, India. Land provision and amenities have been limited. Death rates have increased, food reserves have been depleted and cattle have died[8].

◆ Indigenous people displaced by the Ok Tedi mine in Papua New Guinea have become increasingly reliant on imported rice and tinned fish. Traditional subsistence food growing and trading has been eroded[24].

2.3   MENTAL DISORDER

Displaced peoples often migrate to urban slums where they are disoriented, unsupported, poor and susceptible to alcoholism and prostitution[8].

3   CHANGES IN LAND USE

Land use may change from agricultural production to extractive industries, infrastructure development or industrial processes as well as from one agricultural system to another. Previously unexploited land may have provided natural regulation systems such as flood protection or habitats for predators of agricultural pests and valuable resources for the local population. Natural resource development can effect both the environment and human contact with the environment.

3.1   COMMUNICABLE DISEASE

The abundance of vector breeding sites and the degree of contact between people and vectors may be altered. The abundance of animal host reservoirs may also change.

Land distribution schemes may promote colonization of new lands. Settlers are likely to encounter natural foci of communicable diseases for which they may be ill-prepared. Examples include encounters with leishmaniasis in the steppes of the former USSR and in the forests of South America[26]. In forest areas, the opening of new roads has encouraged an influx of farmers, miners, loggers and others. There have been serious resurgences of malaria concentrated on settlements, mines and periurban areas. New lands are likely to be marginal: in wetter areas they may be forested and in drier areas they may be semi-arid. The pattern of diseases encountered will vary.

EXAMPLE

◆ Opening of new roads and distribution of land in Brazil has encouraged an influx of farmers, miners, loggers and others. There has been a serious resurgence of malaria concentrated on settlements, mines and periurban areas[27].

Deforestation tends to degrade watersheds, leading to increased surface run-off. Erratic stream flows lead to alternate water shortage and flooding. Floods contaminate potable water supplies. Water shortages lead to reliance on contaminated supplies. Both promote waterborne disease transmission.

Changes in land use due to change in agricultural practices, use for mining, construction, reservoirs or road building can remove surface cover and degrade soils. Exposed, dry soils turn into dust bowls. High levels of air-borne dust promote eye and respiratory disease and increased transmission of meningitis[28].

3.2   MALNUTRITION

Many development projects, including mining, farming, forestry, construction, reservoirs and road building activities reduce the land available for the gathering of food, water or fuel.

EXAMPLE

◆ The land irrigated by the Narmada Dam in India may not be as fertile or produce as much food as that lost from the flooded area and the land taken up by canals[8].

Common property resources and forests play a critical role in cushioning the effect of seasonality and food shortage. This role is especially important for the more vulnerable members of communities and households whose entitlements are few. Policies which protect common land strengthen the coping mechanisms of the poor[29]. The very poor, and among them pregnant and lactating women and pre-school children, are especially vulnerable to infectious diseases as a result of bodyweight changes associated with seasonal malnutrition and immunodepression[30].

Loss of natural resources or changes in farming systems may increase the workload of women who are already overworked. The excess work may lead to a negative energy balance and a reduction in their nutritional status. Another consequence is that women may have less time available to care for children or attend at health clinics. The increase in workload can occur in several ways.

Vulnerable subsistence communities depend on unoccupied lands for many of their daily requirements. It is often the duty of women to gather wild food, fuel wood or to collect water. When such land is used for a development project, the community may be deprived of a vital resource. Alternative supplies of that resource may be further away and the workload of women is increased.

Switching land use from subsistence to cash crops can also increase women's workloads. Cash crops may require more work in areas for which women are traditionally responsible, such as weeding.

A change of cropping system may alter the flow of cash into the household. The cash earned may be controlled by men and not used to buy additional food for the family as women would prefer. This may replace a subsistence system in which food is grown and used directly for household consumption. The consequence may be a reduction in family nutrition.

Land tenure, legal access and control over land can have important effects on household income and hence health. Other determinants of household income include improved access to credit, working capital and physical security.

Development schemes have sometimes ignored or suppressed women's land rights, negotiations about land reallocation being conducted with men. In Africa, particularly, loss of land customarily used for subsistence crops has been associated with food scarcity[31].

A wide range of development projects increase the value of farming land, promoting land sales and cash cropping and reducing food security. *See also Forestry, chapter 9.*

3.3   INJURY

Changes in land use may bring an increase in traffic, an increase in contact between people and roads and an associated increase in road traffic injuries. Dwellings or business operations may be established by individuals without any consultation with the authorities. Even planned developments by government departments or development agencies may not go through a consultation process with other departments. Often the relevant technical and planning expertise may be in short supply. Responsibilities in some areas may overlap or be duplicated or there may be no organisation at all responsible. Access ways, buildings and advertising hoardings may then be built too close to the roadway. This creates conflict between pedestrians and traffic. It also creates conflict between stationary, slow moving and fast moving traffic. *See "Towards Safer Roads in Developing Countries"*[32] *and Public Services, chapter 11, Urban Development.*

4 CONSTRUCTION

Many development projects include a construction phase. Large scale construction requires migrant labour (*see section 1*) and may take place in remote rural areas. Small scale construction may use a local labour force, sub-contracted through the informal sector.

Special health services are often provided by construction companies for large projects. Such facilities may or may not be made available to other vulnerable communities, such as resettlers and temporary informal sector residents. The facilities may or may not be integrated into the national health system when the construction phase is completed.

4.1 COMMUNICABLE DISEASE

Construction workers are subject to a range of communicable diseases as a result of migration from different environments or bush clearance activities. Construction camps are notoriously insanitary. The large concentration of single men and a population of camp followers provides a situation of high risk of STD transmission.

EXAMPLES

◆ Malaria outbreaks were avoided during the construction of the following projects by careful planning: the Tungabhadra dam in Andhra Pradesh, India; the hydroelectric plant at Balbina, Amazonas; and the building of the railway from Cuiaba to Porto Velho, Brazil[33,34].

◆ By contrast, in the following projects there were no provisions for malaria control and malaria was a problem: the hydroelectric plant at Tucurui, Brazil; the mining operations at Itaituba and Madeira river, Brazil; the Sakkur barrage in Pakistan; and the Mettur dam in India[35].

4.2 NON-COMMUNICABLE DISEASE

Occupational health and safety are key issues in construction projects. Workloads are heavy and there is often exposure to unsafe noise levels, dust, toxic chemicals, gases, vibration, flammable materials and high temperatures. Much morbidity is work-related rather than occupational: associated with stress, long hours, low pay, poor food, smoking and drinking.

EXAMPLE

◆ In the UK construction industry there are 10 fatalities per 100,000 employees per year. The ratio of major injuries to fatal injuries is 27. Cancers, respiratory and circulatory diseases are more common than in other workers[36].

Occupational diseases of construction workers includes 'white finger'. This follows from extended periods of holding vibrating equipment.

Many women are involved in construction work and the work conditions may increase their vulnerability to spontaneous miscarriage. High mortality rates from injuries and infection have been noted in children living on construction sites[37].

4.3   MALNUTRITION

The nutritional status of poor labourers together with anaemia associated with a parasitic burden, significantly reduce productivity[38,39]. The energy expenditure of heavy labour may exceed energy intake.

EXAMPLE

◆ Smallholders in Kenya were employed on the construction of all-weather rural roads. They laboured in the morning and farmed in the afternoon. Some 62% were male and 38% female. Helminth infection and anaemia were common and 67% were malnourished. The effect of energy food and iron supplementation improved productivity. But many workers used it as a partial substitute for their normal diet. Surprisingly, the nutritional status of women was better than that of the men[39].

4.4   INJURY

The movement of major items of equipment such as turbines, bulldozers and the lorries required to move large amounts of soil and concrete provides major hazards for road users[40].

EXAMPLES

◆ In the construction of the Kainji Dam in Nigeria, road crashes and collisions were the most important cause of death and of major morbidity. Such injuries caused more deaths than all the many communicable disease hazards of the areas[41].

◆ During construction of the Kariba Dam injury accounted for 22 of the 29 deaths among European workers and for 73 out of 122 deaths among Africans. The main causes of death were rock falls, road crashes and collisions and drowning. The percentage of people who reported sick each day varied from 0.5% to 5%. A large percentage of these attenders came with minor injuries which required early treatment to reduce the very real risk of septic complications in the dusty, hot and humid climatic conditions. The frequency of major injuries in an eighteen month period averaged nearly 20 per month. Minor injuries averaged 436 per month in a work force of up to 1,168 Europeans and 6,829 Africans. The relatively low rate of injuries was attributed to training of new labourers and wearing hard hats[40].

---

5   REFERENCES

1   A B Zwi, "Identifying 'high risk situations' for preventing AIDS." *BMJ*. 1991, 303:1527–1529.

2   R M Prothero, and W T S Gould, "Population geography and social provision." in-*Geography and Population, Approaches and Applications*, Ed. J I Clarke . (Pergamon Press, London 1984).

3   R Giel, and J N Van Luijk, "The plight of daily labourers in a coffee growing province of Ethiopia." *Trop Geogr Med*. 1967, 19:304–308.

4   L Levi, "Stress in Industry: Causes, Effects and Prevention." *Occupational Safety and Health Series, vol. 51*, (International Labour Office, Geneva 1984).

5   International Labour Office, "Migrant Workers." (1974) International Labour Conference, 59th Session. vol. VII (1). Geneva. International Labour Office.

6   International Labour Office, "Migrant Workers." (1974) International Labour Conference. vol. VII (2). Geneva. International Labour Office.

7   International Labour Office, "Psychosocial Factors at Work: Recognition and Control." *Occupational Safety and Health Series, vol. 56,* (International Labour Office, Geneva 1986).

8   J C Bhatia, "The Narmada Valley Project." in-*Health Implications of Public Policy, Ed. B Ghosh.* (Indian Institute of Management, Bangalore 1991).

9   C H Browner, "Women, household and health in Latin America." *Soc Sci Med.* 1989, 28:5:461–473.

10 R S Odingo Ed., "An African Dam. Ecological Survey of the Kamburu/Gtaru Hydro-electric Dam Area, Kenya." *Ecological Bulletins.* vol. 29 (Swedish Natural Science Research Council, Stockholm 1979).

11 C W Hunt, "Migrant labour and sexually transmitted disease: AIDS in Africa." *J Hlth Soc Behav.* 1989, 30:December:353–373.

12 F J Bennett, "Gonorrhoea: a rural pattern of transmission." *East Afr Med J.* 1964, 41:4:163–167.

13 A R Verhagen, and W Gemert, "Social and epidemiological determinants of gonorrhoea in an East African country." *Brit J Vener Dis.* 1972, 48:277–286.

14 F J Bennett, "The social determinants of gonorrhoea in an East African town." *East Afr Med J.* 1962, 39:332–336.

15 T D Moodie, "Migrancy and male sexuality on South African gold mines." *J S Afr Stud.* 1989, 14:228–256.

16 R H Meakins, Personal communication.

17 D Wilson, B Sibanda, L Mboyi, and S Msimanga, "A pilot study for an HIV prevention programme among commercial sex workers in Bulawayo, Zimbabwe." *Soc Sci Med.* 1990, 31:609–618.

18 R M Packard, "Industrial production, health and disease in sub-Saharan Africa." *Soc Sci Med.* 1989, 28:5:475–496.

19 A Raikes, "Women's health in East Africa." *Soc Sci Med.* 1989, 28:5:447–459.

20 R H Meakins, "Development, Disease and the Environment." (Robin Press, Lesotho 1981).

21 A I Richards, "Land, Labour and Diet in Northern Rhodesia." (Oxford University Press, Oxford 1939).

22 R W Roundy, "Problems of resettlement and vector-borne diseases associated with dams and other development schemes." in-*Demography and Vector-Borne Diseases, Ed. M W Service .* (CRC Press, Florida 1989).

23 E Colson, "The Social Consequences of Resettlement." (Manchester University Press, Manchester 1971).

24 D Hyndeman, "Ok Tedi: New Guinea's disaster mine." *The Ecologist.* 1988, 18:1:24–29.

25 M H Birley, Personal observation.

26 World Health Organization Commission on Health and Environment, "Our Planet, Our Health." (World Health Organization, Geneva 1992).

27 C E A Coimbra, "Human factors in the epidemiology of malaria in the Brazilian Amazon." *Hum Org.* 1988, 47:3:254–260.

28 B M Greenwood, A K Bradley, I S Blakebrough, and S Wali, "Meningococcal disease and season in sub-saharan Africa." *The Lancet.* 1984, 326:8390:1339–1342.

29 B Agarwal, "Social security and the family: coping with seasonality and calamity in rural India." *J Peasant Stud.* 1990, 17:3:341–412.

30 F Carswell, A O Hughes, R Palmer, J Higginson, P S E G Harland, and R H Meakins, "Nutritional status, globulin titers and parasitic infestations of two populations of Tanzanian school children." *Am J Clin Nutr.* 1981, 43:1292–1299.

31 B Rogers, "The Domestication of Women." (Tavistock Publications Ltd, London 1981).

32 Ross Silcock Partnership, and Overseas Unit of the Transport and Road Research Laboratory, "Towards Safer Roads in Developing Countries. A guide for planners and engineers." 1st ed., (HMSO, 1991).

33 P L Tauil, "Comments on the epidemiology and control of malaria in Brazil." *Mem Inst Oswaldo Cruz.* 1986, 81:supplement 2. Proc. Intern. Symp. on Malaria, Rio de Janiero, Brazil, 1st–5th June 1986:39–41.

34 R B Rao, H R Rao, and B Sundaresan, "Epidemiology of malaria in the Tungabhadra project area of the ceded districts of Madras." *J Mal Inst India.* 1946, 6:323–357.

35 A W A Brown, and J O Deom, "Health aspects of man-made lakes." in-*Man-made Lakes, Their Problems and Environmental Effects, Ed. W C Ackerman, G F White and E B Worthington. Geophysical Monogograph Series No.17.* (American Geophysical Union, Washington D.C. 1973).

36 D Snashall, "Safety and health in the construction industry." *Brit Med J.* 1990, 301:563–564.

37 E R Bhatt, A S Desai, R Thamarajakshi, M Pande, J Arunachalam, and V Kohli, "Shramshakti. Report of the National Commission of Self-employed Women and Women in the Informal Sector." (June 1988) Government of India.

38 R M Brooks, M C Latham, and D W T Crompton, "The relationship of nutrition and health to worker productivity in Kenya." *East Afr Med J.* 1979, 56:6:413–421.

39 J C Wolgemuth, M C Latham, A Hall, A Chesher, and D W T Crompton, "Worker productivity and the nutritional status of Kenyan road construction labourers." *Am J Clin Nutr.* 1982, 36:68–78.

40 M H Webster, "The medical aspects of the Kariba hydro-electric scheme." *Centr Afr J Med.* 1960, 6:supplement:1–36.

41 G Wyatt, Personal communication.

chapter 3

TRANSPORT AND COMMUNICATION

TRANSPORTATION HEALTH HAZARDS AND THE PROJECT STAGE AT WHICH SAFEGUARDS MAY BE REQUIRED

Project stage	Health hazard	Examples and causes
Location	Communicable Disease	Contact with disease foci
	Non-Communicable Disease	Transport and storage of hazardous materials
	Malnutrition	Loss of common property resources, resettlement
Planning and Design	Communicable Disease	Borrow pits, pooling
	Injury	Roads with poor safety features
Construction	Communicable Disease	Poor sanitation, water supply and food hygiene, STDs, exposure to vectors
	Non-Communicable Disease	Inadequate occupational safety measures
	Injury	Inadequate occupational safety measures
Operation	Communicable Disease	Roadside squatters, vector/parasite introductions, waste discharge in ports, STDs associated with transit of single males
	Non-Communicable Disease	Dust, vehicle emissions, noise, transport of hazardous materials
	Injury	Poor vehicle and road maintenance, poor traffic regulation and driver education, increasing vehicle density

1   COMMUNICABLE DISEASE

Road and rail projects built in flat terrain and valley bottoms, especially in areas of seasonally heavy rainfall and clay soils, are often elevated on earthen berms above ground level[1]. Seasonal drainage patterns may be altered or blocked. Such routes built along hillsides, though not elevated above the grade, may block rainfall runoff patterns. Without proper placement of culverts, pooling of water is inevitable. Large volumes of soil extracted during construction create flooded borrow pits. Malaria mosquitoes proliferate in the surface waters and the transmission of malaria may be intensified.

EXAMPLE

◆ Increased malaria has been documented for road construction in the Amazon Basin, Liberia and Kenya. In 1974 some 50% of the malaria in Amazonia was linked to the narrow area of influence of the Trans-amazon Highway[1,2].

Roadside storm water drains in coastal tropical towns and cities are often the sole disposal point for waste. The drains which become blocked by solid waste provide breeding sites for mosquitoes that breed in foul water and transmit filariasis. Spread of parasitic diseases whose ova are passed in excreta is strongly associated with the use of roadside ditches as latrines. The excreta may be washed downstream to nearby moist places or water pools where transmission occurs[3].

EXAMPLE

◆ Filariasis is endemic in coastal Indian towns. As part of a road upgrading programme, curbside L-shaped drains were replaced by deep U-shaped open drains. The new drains were soon filled with rubbish. They were much more difficult to clean out than the old drains and mosquito breeding increased[4].

Unplanned settlements, resthouses, food stalls and garages proliferate along the course of new roads. Often they are situated near ponds where vector mosquitoes and snails breed. The residents of such settlements may have no access to health care facilities. Such informal settlements may serve as a focus for STD transmission by long distance truck drivers and taximen[5,6].

EXAMPLE

◆ A small survey in Uganda in 1986 showed that 68% of women working in bars and 32% of truck drivers were HIV seropositive compared
to 15% of male blood donors and 5% of rural inhabitants. A public
awareness campaign first focused on the main road linking Kenya to
Kampala and Masaka District[5].

By contrast, road improvements can greatly improve access to health
facilities for poor rural communities. Roads simplify the circulation of
health workers improving case finding, treatment and follow-up for communicable disease control such as tuberculosis. They also improve the
response to emergencies such as famine.

EXAMPLE

◆ A study of the impact of a new rural road in Kenya indicated that:
travel fares were reduced due to increased competition between
operators; more visits were made to local health facilities; all communities benefited but the gap between wealthier and poorer
communities was widened. Improved access by the very poor to
free, but more distant, health facilities was an important benefit[7,8].

Road projects enable malaria and other communicable diseases to spread to
previously uninfected areas. Roads change the patterns of human mobility
and circulation, enabling vulnerable people to enter endemic regions.

Workers engaged in the construction of roads or laying of telephone lines
through undisturbed countryside may contact natural disease foci. An
example would be scrub typhus in Southeast Asia.

Seaports are a traditional focus for STD transmission associated with sailors,
military personnel and tourists[9].

EXAMPLE

◆ A survey in Manila found that 5 out of 6 people seropositive for HIV
were sex workers connected to military bases[9].

Air travel provides an ideal opportunity for insect disease vectors to migrate
to new regions unless strict disinfection measures are maintained. However,
the recent spread of the Asian tiger mosquito into the USA is attributed to
used tyre imports.

2   NON-COMMUNICABLE DISEASE

Many roads in rural areas are unpaved and some are used primarily for the short term extraction of natural resources. The large volumes of dust disturbed by traffic on unpaved roads may be a cause of respiratory disease[10].

EXAMPLE

◆ In the Appalachian states of the USA many people live by unpaved roads. Dust particle levels are unacceptably high within 100m of the roadside and they may aggravate pre-existing respiratory disease[10].

Motor vehicles are the largest single source of several important air pollutants[11] (See also Energy, chapter 5, Fossil Fuels). There are over 500M vehicles on roads in the world and the annual growth rate averages 3%. Heavy duty trucks and buses are an increasingly important proportion of the total. The emissions contribute to eye irritation, headaches, heart disease, upper respiratory illness, asthma and reduced pulmonary function. Lead pollution may affect the neurological development of children and the consequences may extend into adulthood. The problem could easily be solved, at least in part, by the use of unleaded petrol in engines[12]. Technologies are available to reduce emissions cost-effectively. Fuel quality is an important determinant. The increase in number of vehicles offsets the beneficial effect of emission control. Noise pollution is an associated problem.

EXAMPLE

◆ Exposure of 'jeepney' drivers in Manila to total suspended matter, carbon monoxide, sulphur dioxide and lead was above WHO and national air quality standards. The prevalence of chronic respiratory symptoms, chronic obstructive airway disease and reduced lung function was significantly higher than in commuters. Smoking was a contributory factor[13].

---

3   MALNUTRITION

Roads built on valley floors may reduce the availability of agricultural land and increase roadside land values. Food prices may rise and food security may decrease.

4 INJURY

There appears to be a strong link between development and motor-vehicle related mortality[14]. Road injury fatality rates per licensed vehicle are often 20 to 30 times as high as those in European countries[15], and the rate has worsened over the past decade[16]. It is well accepted nowadays that injuries are no accident. They are predictable, avoidable and amenable to public health intervention[17].

Of 500,000 to 856,000 fatalities from automobile crashes and collisions globally per year, about 350,000 to 637,000 are in developing countries where the number of motor vehicles relative to the population are generally much lower than in developed countries. Two thirds of the crashes and collisions involve pedestrians, mostly children, and two thirds occur in cities or surrounding areas. There are ten to twenty times as many people injured as killed. It is mostly young people who are killed or disabled. The loss of productivity and the cost of treatment and future support is considerable to a developing country. In the age group 5–44 years, automobile crashes and collisions are the second most important cause of death in the world[12,18].

EXAMPLES

◆ One unpublished report tried to identify the financial savings attributable to road upgrading projects by including substantial sums to reflect pain, grief and suffering from traffic crashes and collisions[19].

◆ Traffic crashes and collisions in Papua New Guinea were estimated to cost 1% of GNP in 1978[20].

◆ Between 1968 and 1985 the number of deaths from vehicle crashes increased by over 300% in African countries and by over 170% in Asian countries. In developed countries in the same period, the number of deaths declined by 25%[15].

Fatality rates appear to reduce with increasing vehicle ownership, apparently as a result of behaviour modification[19]. Fatality rates per person injured improve significantly with increasing medical facilities. Hospitals near main routes may have most surgical beds occupied by road crash/collision victims who have to remain for extended periods. Traffic related injuries may pose a great financial burden on the health service.

Road users frequently disobey road signs and markings. This is due in part to lack of knowledge of safety rules and regulations and lack of concentration due to tiredness or use of stimulant drugs. Poor maintenance and gross over-loading of vehicles are common. Commercial and public service vehicles constitute a larger percentage of road collisions in developing countries than in developed. Pedestrians, cyclists and slow moving vehicles are particularly at risk[15]. Rates of crashes/collisions are also associated with the quality of highway engineering[19]. High benefit-cost ratios have been demonstrated in developed countries from low cost remedial measures. See "Towards Safer Roads in Developing Countries. A guide for planners and engineers"[15] for more information.

EXAMPLES

◆ It is estimated that 15–18% of drivers in Bangladesh, The Ivory Coast and Nigeria are under-age and 60% have not passed a driving test[21].

◆ In Indian cities, buses are involved in around 25% of all injury incidents while the equivalent figure for Britain is under 4%[15].

◆ Commercial vehicle occupants in Kenya contribute to 16% of all road collision casualties while the figure for most developed countries is under 5%[15].

◆ A study of traffic related injuries in one area of Egypt found that 67% occurred in towns, 33% in rural areas; 54% of injuries to pedestrians occurred in towns but villages through which highways pass are also highly dangerous. The weather played a larger role in rural areas and on highways than in towns: fog and rain were obvious causes of many crashes[22].

There are opportunities to improve safety. For example, open-backed vehicles used for passenger transport are a major source of transport injuries in Papua New Guinea. Import duties favour these in place of safer enclosed vehicles[23]. A survey indicated that only about 10% of front-seat car occupants in PNG wore seat-belts[24]. Stresses on drivers, especially of trucks and buses, may be exacerbated by their methods of payment. Many of them are paid by the number of trips which they do in a specified period of time, or by the distances they cover. They therefore have an incentive to drive fast, to use stimulants such as caffeine and various drugs and not to rest even if they feel tired.

New and upgraded roads create a particular hazard for pedestrians. Very often rural people have no experience of fast moving traffic. They may wander across unfenced roads sometimes driving herds of animals. They may have no conception of the sort of distance required for a fast moving vehicle to come to a stop.

The importance of alcohol as a causal factor of road vehicle related injuries is recognised but few figures are available for developing countries. Alcohol is increasingly used and promoted, partly as a consequence of the development process.

EXAMPLES

◆ The road from Lagos to Ibadan in Nigeria was notorious as a traffic hazard since it was poorly constructed and had insufficient capacity for the rapidly growing traffic flows. Badly damaged lorries and cars were to be found at almost every narrow bridge and littered along the roadside. When a new motorway was constructed traffic speeds were greatly increased. The motorway was unfenced for most of its length and villagers, laden with firewood, crossed the road between the rapidly moving vehicles. The number of road injuries among pedestrians increased[25].

◆ A Zimbabwe survey showed that over 50% of drivers and over 70% of pedestrians killed in road traffic "accidents" had alcohol in their blood.

◆ Among hospitalised casualties resulting from motor-cycle crashes in Delhi, 29% admitted having consumed alcohol before the crash[26].

---

5 REFERENCES

1 S K Ault, "Effect of demographic patterns, social structure, and human behaviour on malaria." in-*Demography and Vector-Borne Diseases*, Ed. M W Service. (CRC Press, Florida 1989).

2 C E A Coimbra, "Human factors in the epidemiology of malaria in the Brazilian Amazon." *Hum Org.* 1988, 47:3:254–260.

3 R H Meakins, Personal communication.

4 M H Birley, Personal observation.

5 J W Carswell, "HIV infections in healthy persons in Uganda." *AIDS.* 1987, 1:223–227.

6 O P Arya, A O Osoba, and F T Bennett, "Tropical Venereology: Medicine in the Tropics." 2nd ed., (Churchill Livingstone, London 1988).

7 T Airey, "The influence of road construction on the health care behaviour of rural households in the Meru district of Kenya." *Transport Reviews.* 1991, 11:3:273–290.

8 J Howe, "Evaluation of the Thuchi-Nkubu Road, Kenya." (June 1989) Overseas Development Administration. EV 267.

9 The Panos Institute, "Aids and the Third World." (The Panos Institute, London 1988).

10 E N Howze, and J M Hughes, "Elevated respirable dust levels along unpaved coal-haul roads: a rural public health problem." *Am Rev of Resp Dis Part 2.* 1990, 141:4:A77.

11 M P Walsh, "The Impact of Transport on Health and the Environment: a Background Paper." (1991) World Health Organization Commission on Health and Environment. (unpublished).

12 World Health Organization Commission on Health and Environment, "Our Planet, Our Health." (World Health Organization, Geneva 1992).

13 R D Subida, and E B Torres, "Epidemiology of Chronic Respiratory Symptoms and Illnesses Among Jeepney Drivers, Air-conditioned Bus Drivers and Commuters Exposed to Vehicular Emissions in Metro Manila, 1990–1991." (November 1991) World Health Organization.

14 G Wintemute, "Is motor vehicle related mortality a disease of development?" *Accid Anal Prev.* 1985, 17:223–237.

15 Ross Silcock Partnership, and Overseas Unit of the Transport and Road Research Laboratory, "Towards Safer Roads in Developing Countries. A guide for planners and engineers." 1st ed., (HMSO, 1991).

16 G D Jacobs, and C A Cutting, "Further research on accident rates in developing countries." *Accid Anal & Prev.* 1986, 18:2:119–127.

17 A Zwi, B Msika, and E Smetannikov, "Causes and remedies." *World Health.* 1993, 46:1:18–20.

18 World Bank, "World Development Report 1993." (Oxford University Press, New York 1993).

19 G D Jacobs, "Road accident prevention: work of the overseas unit, TRRL." (1986) Department of Transport Ed., Sino-British Highways and Urban Traffic Conference. Beijing, China. UK Department of Transport.

20 J D J Havard, "World Health Organization Assignment Report." (1978) World Health Organization Regional Office for the Western Pacific. ICP/HSD/015.

21 World Health Organization, "New approaches to Improve Road Safety." (1989) World Health Organization. Technical Report Series No. 781.

22 I G Badran, "Accidents in the developing world." *World Health.* 1993, 46:1:14–15.

23 D C Nelson, and J V Strueber, "The effect of open-back vehicles on casualty rates: the case of Papua New Guinea." *Accid Anal & Prev.* 1991, 23:2/3:109–117.

24 J A Lourie, "Use of seat-belts in Port Moresby." *Papua New Guinea Med J.* 1982, 25:4:214–218.

25 G Wyatt, Personal communication.

26 A Zwi, "The public health burden of injury in developing countries: a critical review of the literature." *Trop Dis Bull.* 1993, 90:4:R5–R45.

chapter 4

MINING HEALTH HAZARDS AND THE PROJECT STAGE AT WHICH SAFEGUARDS MAY BE REQUIRED

Project stage	Health hazard	Examples and causes
Location	Communicable Disease	Contact with disease foci
	Non-Communicable Disease	Pollution from spoil heaps
	Malnutrition	Loss of common property resources
Planning and Design	Non-Communicable Disease	Dust-induced lung disease
Construction	Communicable Disease	Poor sanitation, water supply and food hygiene, STDs, exposure to vectors
	Non-Communicable Disease	Inadequate occupational safety measures
	Injury	Inadequate occupational safety measures
Operation	Communicable Disease	Respiratory disease, contact with disease foci, STDs
	Non-Communicable Disease	Respiratory disease, pollution from spoil deposits and tailing dams, noise
	Injury	Structural failure, flooding, explosion, road haulage, abandoned mine workings

See also Cross-Cutting Issues, chapter 2, Changes in Land Use, and Labour Mobility, and Manufacture and Trade, chapter 12, Occupational Health Hazards of Industry.

1   COMMUNICABLE DISEASE

Opencast mineworks have often been responsible for increased malaria transmission, during the different project phases from land clearing to operation. Mineral wealth is often located in remote areas, such as forests, where labourers may be exposed to disease vectors. In some cases the vectors are associated with forest shade and in other cases they proliferate when the shade is removed by partial clearing.

Mining often requires large quantities of water. Dams and canals are created to pump water in or out of the mine workings. Dumping of tailings creates artificial lakes and marshes and abandoned workings become flooded[2,3]. These water bodies may support vector breeding.

The spread of epidemic diseases like AIDS poses a particular threat to such industries. This has been recognised on Zambia's copperbelt.

The circulation of labour associated with mining may transport new diseases both into and out of the mining region.

EXAMPLES

◆ A gold-rush in Brazil during 1985 brought non-immune migrants from neighbouring states to a malaria endemic district. Of the malaria cases recorded some 49% came from areas of mining activity[1].

◆ In India, the mining of minerals and coal and the production of oil have been notoriously affected by malaria. In 1933 malaria brought iron and magnesium mines to a standstill in Orissa[1].

◆ Tin extraction in Maniema, Eastern Zaire, was initially based on alluvial deposits. Schistosomiasis and its vector snail were absent. When extraction shifted to primary veins large quantities of water were required. Numerous dams and canals were constructed. The vector and the disease spread rapidly wherever the calcium content of the water was relatively high. However, even in villages with 100% prevalence, the intensity of infection had not reduced the work capacity of the labourers[2].

◆ In Guyana, large scale mining operations caused outbreaks of malaria when infected miners returned home[4].

2 NON-COMMUNICABLE DISEASE

The air-borne particulate matter associated with mining leads to irreversible lung damage and respiratory disease.

The health impacts of deep-rock mining by migrant labour in Southern Africa has been well documented. Chronic lung disease is common and this often reactivates latent tuberculosis and increases susceptibility to infectious pneumonias that are exported to the labour reserve[5,6]. Such occupational diseases are often not recorded or recognised in regions where compensation payments would be compulsory.

EXAMPLE

◆ In the South African mines the incidence of tuberculosis has risen dramatically over the last decade to a rate of 800–1000 per 100,000[7].

Communities living near mines frequently suffer from chronic exposure to heavy metals such as lead[8], cadmium[9], arsenic[10], copper and uranium[11]. The wastewater discharge and groundwater associated with mineworks is often heavily contaminated with soluble metal salts. Metal compounds contaminate waste tips and surface soils. Symptoms of intoxication include behavioral changes, nausea and headache, reproductive failure[12], foetal damage and various cancers. Women are more susceptible than men to the toxic effects of lead[13].

Coal tips pose health hazards of fires, slides and water impoundment. If the waste ignites, gaseous emissions can contain carbon monoxide, carbon dioxide, hydrogen sulphide, sulphur dioxide and ammonia. These can damage human health directly and damage trees and crops[15].

The incidence of lung cancer is increased by underground mining. The main factor is believed to be exposure to radon, a radioactive gas[16]. Asbestos may be extremely hazardous not only to the workers involved with mining and processing it, but also to their families and other communities in the vicinity of asbestos mines and processing plants, as dust may be brought home on clothes.

EXAMPLES

◆ Lead mines in Anambra State, Nigeria, have caused widespread lead poisoning[11].

◆ Children in a Canadian mining community had significantly elevated blood lead levels[8].

◆ Residents of a USA mining community were exposed to lead and cadmium. The prevalence of kidney and heart diseases and skin cancer was significantly elevated[9].

◆ Former Japanese mine workers suffering from chronic arsenic poisoning had a significantly elevated cancer rate[10].

◆ Pollution from Ok Tedi mine, Papua New Guinea, has threatened rivers, food crops and fish used by 40,000 people. In 1988, suspended sediments and heavy metals were said to have exceeded US standards by 10,000 per cent[14].

---

3 MALNUTRITION

Mining requires land and water and produces large quantities of solid and liquid waste. Substantial areas of agricultural land are lost from productive agriculture. Local subsistence farmers and fishing communities lose their food supplies and rates of malnutrition may increase. *See also Cross-Cutting Issues, chapter 2, Changes in Land Use.*

4 INJURY

Opencast mining requires the use of very heavy vehicles and the transport of minerals and soil over long distances. The combination of heavy and light vehicles with pedestrians on roads may lead to a high risk of crashes and collisions.

The high levels of traumatic injury among mineworkers is sometimes associated with an absence of labour organisations capable of negotiating for improved safety. In many countries there are women mineworkers who may face special hazards while being paid less[17].

EXAMPLES

◆ In Bolivia the population of 24,000 large mine workers had 5,430 injuries in 1972[18].

◆ Noise induced hearing loss is reported in Zambian copper mine workers. It is proportional to the numbers of years exposed[19]. Many miners never used ear protection.

Quarry and deep mine workers suffer problems of heat stroke. Eye injuries result from alloy and stone chips. Other injuries may result from falling rock, slippery surfaces, flooding and exposure to electrical current. Ear protection and helmets may be very hot and uncomfortable in deep mines: it is not surprising that workers sometimes fail to use such personal protective equipment even when it is made available to them.

EXAMPLE

◆ In construction of the Bougainville Copper mine in Papua New Guinea, a peak labour force of 4,000 expatriates and 6,000 Papua New Guineans was involved. 16 miles of mountain road, two small towns and a port were required. 40 million tons of waste rock were removed before mining began. Vehicle crashes were the most important cause of deaths among the workforce[20].

Extractive industries all involve the use of heavy machinery and workers are subjected to high noise levels. The petroleum industry exposes workers to high noise levels from drills, compressors, motors, blowers, generators, pumps and valves[21].

EXAMPLE

◆ A study of South African mine-workers who were left permanently disabled following mine "accidents" indicated that compensation payments were lower than poverty datum levels and that high rates of inflation rapidly eroded their value. Compensation did not redress the income loss that these workers experienced. In 1986, 800 miners died and 12,700 had injuries severe enough to be notified in terms of South African legislation[22].

Abandoned open caste mines usually involve slimy depressions which accumulate water. In Jos, Nigeria, the abandoned old tin workings were often used as a water source. They were associated with a high death rate. Children especially slipped on the clays while drawing water, became entrapped in the pools and drowned[23].

5 REFERENCES

1 M W Service, Personal communication.
2 A M Polderman, Kayiteshonga Mpamila, J P Manshande, B Gryseels, and O van Schayk, "Historical, geological and ecological aspects of transmission of intestinal schistosomiasis in Maniema, Kivu Province, Zaire." *Ann Soc Belge Méd Trop.* 1985, 65:251–261.

3 J H van Ee, and A M Polderman, "Physiological performance and work capacity of tin mine labourers infested with schistosomiasis in Zaire." *Trop Geogr Med.* 1984, 36:259–266.
4 G Giglioli, "Ecological change as a factor in renewed malaria transmission in an eradicated area." *WHO Bull.* 1963, 29:131–145.
5 Zwi, S Marks, and N Andersson, "Health, apartheid and the frontline states." *Soc Sci Med.* 1988, 27:7:661–665.
6 I M Phimister, "African labour conditions in the southern Rhodesia mining industry." *Centr Afr J Med.* 1976, 21 and 22:214–220; 63–68,173–181,224–249.
7 R M Packard, "Industrial production, health and disease in sub-Saharan Africa." *Soc Sci Med.* 1989, 28:5:475–496.
8 L Chenard, F Turcotte, and S Cordier, "Lead absorption by children living near a primary copper smelter." *Can J Pub Hlth.* 1987, 78:5:295–298.
9 J S Neuberger, M Mulhall, M C Pomatto, J Sheverbush, and R S Hassanein, "Health problems in Galena, Kansas: a heavy metal mining superfund site." *Sci Total Environ.* 1990, 94:3:261–272.
10 T Tsuda, T Nagira, M Yamamoto, and Y Kume, "An epidemiological study on cancer in certified arsenic poisoning patients in Toroku." *Ind Health.* 1990, 28:2:53–62.
11 B C E Egboka, G I Nwankwor, I P Orajaka, and A O Ejiofor, "Principles and problems of environmental pollution of groundwater resources with case examples from developing countries." *Environ Hlth Perspect.* 1989, 83:39–68.
12 Anonymous, "Lead poisoning decreases male sex function; causes LH defect." *Ob Gyn News.* 1977, 12:24:5.
13 W N Rom, "Effects of lead on the female and reproduction: a review." *Mount Sinai J Med.* 1976, 43:5:542–552.
14 D Hyndeman, "Ok Tedi: New Guinea's disaster mine." *The Ecologist.* 1988, 18:1:24–29.
15 J A Lee, "The Environment, Public Health and Human Ecology: Considerations for Economic Development." (John Hopkins University Press, Baltimore 1985).
16 B Nemery, "Metal toxicity and the respiratory tract." *Eur Respir J.* 1990, 3:2:202–219.
17 E R Bhatt, A S Desai, R Thamarajakshi, M Pande, J Arunachalam, and V Kohli, "Shramshakti. Report of the National Commission of Self-employed Women and Women in the Informal Sector." (June 1988) Government of India.
18 M A El-Batawi, "Special problems of occupational health in the developing countries." in-*Occupational Health Practice, Ed. R S F Schilling.* 2nd ed., (Butterworths, London 1981).
19 M N Obiako, "Deafness and the mining industry in Zambia." *East Afr Med J.* 1979, 56:9:445–449.
20 G Wyatt, Personal communication.
21 World Health Organization Commission on Health and Environment, "Our Planet, Our Health." (World Health Organization, Geneva 1992).
22 J P Leger, and R S Arkles, "Permanent disability in black mineworkers. A critical analysis." *South African Medical Journal,* 1989, 76:557–561.
23 R H Meakins, Personal communication.

chapter 5

ENERGY SECTOR HEALTH HAZARDS AND THE PROJECT STAGE AT WHICH SAFEGUARDS MAY BE REQUIRED

Project stage	Health hazard	Examples and causes
Location	Communicable Disease	Contact with disease foci, pollution of water sources
	Non-Communicable Disease	Air and water pollution
	Malnutrition	Loss of common property resources
	Injury	Fire, explosion, road haulage, earthquake
Planning and Design	Communicable disease	Resettlement, access roads, excreta disposal
	Non-Communicable Disease	Air and water pollution
	Malnutrition	Resettlement
	Injury	Road haulage, structural faults
Construction	Communicable Disease	Poor sanitation, water supply and food hygiene, STDs, exposure to vectors
	Non-Communicable Disease	Inadequate occupational safety measures
	Injury	Inadequate occupational safety measures
Operation	Communicable Disease	Creation of vector breeding sites by draw-down and stream ponding
	Non-Communicable Disease	Air pollution, smoke, fly ash and leachate disposal, exposure to electromagnetic fields, noise and vibration
	Malnutrition	Fuel crops replace food crops
	Injury	Road traffic crashes and collisions, domestic burns and scalds, fuel leaks, illegal connection, structural failure

Provision of energy has many direct and indirect benefits to health. For example: electricity is used in refrigeration for vaccines and fossil fuel is used in fertilizer manufacture to enable increased food production.

There are three recent major reviews of the negative health impacts of the energy sector[1,2,3]. This review focuses on fossil fuels, biomass fuels, geothermal energy and hydropower. Nuclear power is not included because the health hazards are already widely discussed.

The WHO World Commission on Health and the Environment identified the following four priority areas for immediate action[3]:

◆ Indoor air pollution from biomass and coal combustion;

◆ Exposure of large urban populations to high levels of ambient air pollution;

◆ Serious injuries associated with extraction, storage and power generation;

◆ Global climate change (*outside the scope of this review*).

1   FOSSIL FUELS

1.1   NON-COMMUNICABLE DISEASE

Fossil fuels (coal, gas, and oil) account for most of the global industrial energy sources. The health hazards of fossil fuel use can be classified according to time of onset of the potential illness or disability or according to the stage in the fossil fuel cycle. See Table 1. The long term mutagenic and carcinogenic effects are the most serious and most uncertain.

The pollutants emitted by the combustion of fossil fuels have an impact on the health of nearby communities and are also dispersed over large areas. They include sulphur dioxide, nitrogen dioxide, carbon monoxide, particulate matter, ash and carbon dioxide. Carbon monoxide accumulates in buildings when combustion chambers and exhaust ducts are not properly

---

EXAMPLES

◆ In London, 1952, when the atmospheric concentration of sulphur dioxide and suspended particles exceeded 1000 ug/m^3 the total daily mortality rate doubled. Similar effects have been reported from Japan[4].

◆ A rapid increase in upper respiratory infection was reported in the vicinity of a new coal-fired power station at Batangaas, Philippines[5].

◆ In China, burning high fluoride content coals contributes to endemic fluorosis affecting large populations[6].

TABLE I   Health hazards associated with the fossil fuel cycle (Modified from World Health Organization[2]).

Classification according to time of onset of illness or disability

Health hazard	Acute	Intermediate	Long-term
Vehicle crashes and collisions	✓		
Fires and explosions	✓		
Work injuries	✓		
Eye irritation	✓		
Respiratory tract irritation and impairment	✓		
Aggravation of respiratory and cardiovascular conditions	✓	✓	
Neurophysiological impairment	✓		
Odour and noise	✓		
Psychological effects	✓		
Skin irritation	✓		
Specific acute toxicity	✓		
Effect of organic and inorganic pollutants		✓	
Effects on human reproduction		✓	
Carcinogenicity			✓
Mutagenicity			✓
Consequences for health of ecological damage			✓

TABLE I   continued

Categories of health hazard and stage in the fossil fuel cycle

Fuel cycle	Injuries	Diseases	Cancers	Genetic
Raw materials	✔			
Exploration	✔			
Mining, extraction	✔	✔	✔	✔
Processing, preparation	✔	✔		
Storage	✔	✔		
Distribution	✔		✔	
Small-scale end-use	✔	✔	✔	✔
Industrial end-use	✔	✔	✔	✔
Transport, excl. traffic crashes and collisions	✔	✔	✔	✔
Waste disposal	✔	✔	✔	✔
Decommissioning	✔			

Definite or major effects ✔
Potential or lesser effects ✔

sealed. It impedes oxygen transport in the human body leading to neurological, physiological and cardiovascular impairment. Nitrogen dioxide impedes respiration. Oxides of nitrogen react with hydrocarbons to produce photochemical smog that causes eye irritation and acute respiratory disease.

High concentrations of sulphur dioxide and particulates increase respiratory disease and can increase mortality. Hydrogen sulphide exposure is an occupational hazard and in high concentrations causes acute intoxication and eye ailments ('gas eye')[7].

EXAMPLE

◆ In Mexico, 1950, an oilfield flare malfunctioned releasing hydrogen sulphide; 320 people were hospitalised and 22 died[7].

The relative health risks of coal- versus oil-based electricity generation are complex. The occupational risks of deep coal mining are well established and include injuries and respiratory disease. *See Mining, chapter 4.* The by-products of coal and oil processing include chemicals that can cause skin tumours and dermatitis. The ash residue from coal burning contains concentrated toxins such as heavy metals. The emissions from coal-fired plants are harder to contain than those from oil-fired power stations. Small to medium sized power stations are more dangerous to the immediate population than large ones because they have lower stacks.

The emissions from petrol or diesel engines are an important source of air-borne pollutants and contribute to photochemical smog.

Urban air pollution from burning fossil fuels regularly exceeds the health-related guidelines established by WHO in over half of the cities that are monitored[3].

EXAMPLE

◆ Burning domestic fuel generates about half of Delhi's air pollution, according to one estimate[8].

Some cities in Central and Southern Africa suffer from thermal inversion smogs made worse by the extensive use of wood and coal for domestic purposes. In Southern Africa this is associated with the spread of tuberculosis and other respiratory diseases[9].

1.2 INJURY

Noise and vibration are occupational hazards of power plants that affect general well-being, hearing and vision.

The transportation of fuel by road and rail increases the risk of traffic crashes and collisions. Fires and explosions are hazards of fuel combustion in power stations. Burns and scalds may occur at various stages of the process.

EXAMPLES

◆ Workers at the Cebu power plant, Philippines, were exposed to noise levels of 102dBA, which was above the permissible limit set by the Department of Labour and Employment[10].

◆ Gas pipeline explosions killed 508 people in Sao Paulo, Brazil in 1984 and 58 people in Mexico in 1978[11]. Gas released in a tank explosion in Mexico in 1984, left 452 dead, over 4,000 injured, and 300,000 required to be evacuated[12].

---

2 BIOMASS FUELS

Biomass fuels are the primary fuel for most domestic users in poor communities. They include wood, logging wastes, animal dung and crop residues. There are important health hazards associated with the collection and burning of biomass.

EXAMPLE

◆ Biomass fuels are used to meet the energy needs of nearly half the world population[8].

2.1 NON-COMMUNICABLE DISEASE/INJURY

Exposure to smoke causes respiratory and eye irritation and associated diseases such as:

◆ Chronic obstructive lung disease;

◆ Heart disease, especially cor pulmonale;

◆ Acute respiratory infections, particularly in children;

◆ Low birth weight due to maternal exposure which is associated with a range of perinatal and infant ill-health;

◆ Eye disorders: conjunctivitis, blindness;

◆ Cancers: lung cancer due to long term exposure to smoke[13,14].

Women and infants are the most vulnerable groups. Household cooking on an open fire has been described as the largest single occupational health problem of women in the world[8,15].The development and utilization of improved cooking-stoves will reduce this health risk and the associated problem of fuel scarcity[16].

EXAMPLES

◆ Biomass stoves are often at floor level causing injuries, especially burns to children, and jeopardizing food hygiene[8].

◆ A study in Nepal in 1986 indicated that improved cooking-stoves were effective in reducing the cook's exposure to health damaging particulates by approximately two thirds. They also reduced carbon monoxide concentrations in kitchens by three-quarters in comparison to neighbouring kitchens with traditional cooking-stoves[17].

Occupational health hazards are identified with long and exhausting journeys bearing heavy fuel loads. *See Forestry, chapter 9.*

2.2   MALNUTRITION

Fuels are produced by the fermentation of food crops such as sugar cane, cassava, corn and sweet sorghum. Sugar cane is the most efficient in terms of net energy yield. The large scale use of such crops to produce fuel could seriously deplete the food supply in local communities. Even crop residues could be more valuable to local farmers as a soil conditioner than fuel produced from the residues. Removal of large quantities of biomass from a given locality will produce changes in soil and aquatic biota that could adversely affect the productivity of fisheries and farms[18].

3   GEOTHERMAL ENERGY

3.1   NON-COMMUNICABLE DISEASE

Geothermal steam tapped from depths of 3,000m carries dirt, impurities, hydrogen sulphide and radon-222, a radioactive gas. Significant quantities of toxic elements, such as arsenic, chromium, copper and mercury, accumulate in the sludge[19]. The sludge may be discharged into rivers and accumulate in the fish food chain. Exposure to non-condensing gases is the most serious public and occupational health concern[20].

3.2   INJURY

The hazards of drilling geothermal sources include violent explosions and emissions of large quantities of hydrogen sulphide.

4   HYDROPOWER

There are important health hazards associated with the large bodies of surface water that are stored, diverted and discharged during construction and operation of dams.

Large dam developments may not take account of health in the calculation of cost-benefit ratios. Smaller projects may produce the same or higher levels of benefit for less cost to health.

EXAMPLE

◆   The Narmada Dam, India, may have a negative cost-benefit ratio if the costs of loss of forests, which provide subsistence for thousands of people, are included[21].

The health of the often large numbers of people who must be resettled is an important cause for concern. *See Resettlement, chapter 2 section 2.*

4.1 COMMUNICABLE DISEASE

The communicable diseases most often associated with hydropower are malaria, schistosomiasis and onchocerciasis.

Large engineering projects involving rivers have frequently led to explosive malaria epidemics during construction. The main cause is the increase in water-filled excavations and diversions.

EXAMPLE

◆ The diversion of the Thenpennai River for a 10 km stretch near the Sathanur Dam, Tamil Nadu, exposed a rocky river bed in which mosquitoes could breed. There was a resurgence of malaria[22].

Mosquitoes which transmit malaria often breed in the shallow, sheltered margins of reservoirs[23]. However, there is much variation between regions. In Africa, malaria mosquito breeding is also associated with drawdown that exposes numerous puddles on gently sloping shores. In Asia, downstream pools in the river bed tend to be more important.

EXAMPLE

◆ A small dam was built to regulate flow to the Edea hydroelectric plant in Cameroon. The shallow waters contain abundant vegetation and larvae of the mosquito *Anopheles funestus*. The prevalence of *falciparum* malaria is high in surrounding villages and decreases with distance from the lake[23].

Schistosomiasis and, to a lesser extent, dracunculiasis are commonly reported hazards of reservoir construction. The large reservoirs usually associated with hydropower have many sheltered, shallow inlets where aquatic vegetation thrives. Informal settlements of fishers are frequently a vulnerable group.

An increase in schistosomiasis has been observed simultaneously across the whole of Africa where water development has taken place. The increases in prevalence have often been dramatic and the intense haematuria in children has caused public alarm[24]. By contrast, in Asia schistosomiasis is contained within small endemic foci and dam development has often proceeded without outbreaks of the disease.

EXAMPLE

◆ Urinary schistosomiasis was locally of low prevalence before the Akosombo Dam was built in Ghana. The reservoir attracted some 150,000 lakeside residents and there was an explosive increase in prevalence. Prevalence rates fell rapidly with distance from the lake shore due to decreasing dependence of the lake for water needs[24].

In South-east Asia and countries of the former USSR *Opisthorchis* infection (human liver fluke) is associated with reservoir construction[8].

Water outflow from large hydropower schemes is often erratic or polluted. Erratic downstream flows promote stream pool breeding of mosquito vectors while spillways, in some regions, support breeding of black fly vectors of river blindness.

EXAMPLE

◆ The natural flow in the upper reaches of the Mahaweli river, Sri Lanka, was interrupted by dams and diversions. Stream pools formed in the dry river-bed in which malaria vectors bred. A reservoir of infection was created by human circulation between lowland resettlement sites and riverine villages[25].

There is a possible connection between the epidemic of visceral leishmaniasis in southern Sudan that has killed 30,000 and the construction of the Owen Falls Dam some 1,000 km upstream 25 years previously. It has been suggested that the altered water regime caused widespread flooding in Sudan that destroyed the closed canopy woodland and created breeding sites for the vector[26].

Reservoir outflow is often polluted by decomposing plant material. Pollution reduces access to potable water for downstream communities that rely on the river, promoting transmission of waterborne diseases. Reduced stream flows alter the replenishment rate of aquifers, affecting domestic water supply, and promoting saline intrusion on to irrigated lands. Reduced nutrient flows disrupt fisheries and reduce food security.

EXAMPLE

◆ Groundwater rose in Lower Egypt as a result of the Aswan Dam. Wastewater disposal was disrupted and aquifers became polluted[27].

4.2   INJURY

The direct risks of hydropower are largely concerned with the traumatic injury associated with large construction projects. *See Cross-Cutting Issues, chapter 2, Construction.*

The risks of failure of dams have been reviewed by the World Bank[28].

There is concern over the effects of reservoirs on the risks of earthquakes. The Narmada Dam in India is being constructed in an area classified as having moderate seismicity with infrequent occurrence of earthquakes[21].

Drowning is a major cause of death in a variety of developing countries, including China. It is the fourth leading cause of injury death in Zimbabwe: increasing the number of reservoirs and dams may increase the levels of contact which people, especially children, have with these water masses, and may therefore increase the number of drowning and near drowning episodes.

5   TRANSMISSION LINES

5.1   NON-COMMUNICABLE DISEASE

There is current concern about the effects of electromagnetic radiation from high tension power lines, but little conclusive information. Exposure to electromagnetic fields may increase the risk of some cancers, in particular leukaemia, lymphoma and nervous system tumours[8].

5.2   INJURY

There are reported cases of electrocution among workers in contact with metal pipes which have become live through unintentional contact with power lines[29].

In Zimbabwe there have been anecdotal accounts of rural farmers being electrocuted after attempting to divert electricity sources to create electrified fences to protect their cattle from theft.

6   REFERENCES

1 D E C Cooper Weil, A P Alicbusan, J F Wilson, M R Reich, and D J Bradley, "The Impact of Development Policies on Health: A Review of the Literature." (World Health Organization, Geneva 1990).

2 World Health Organization, "Health Impact of Different Energy Sources. A Challenge for the End of the Century." (1983) World Health Organization Working Group on Health and Energy in Europe. European Series No.19.

3 World Health Organization Commission on Health and Environment, "Report of the Panel on Energy." (World Health Organization, Geneva 1992).

4 World Health Organization, "Sulphur Oxides and Suspended Particulate Matter." (1979) World Health Organization. Environmental Health Criteria No. 8.

5 Environmental Management Bureau (Philippines), "The Philippine Environment of the Eighties." (Department of Environment and Natural Resources, Manila 1990).

6 PEPAS, "Summary of Activities." (1991) World Health Organisation, Pacific Regional Centre for the Promotion of Environmental Planning and Applied Studies.

7 World Health Organization, "Hydrogen Sulphide." (1981) World Health Organization. Environmental Health Criteria No.19.

8 World Health Organization Commission on Health and Environment, "Our Planet, Our Health." (World Health Organization, Geneva 1992).

9 R H Meakins, "Development, Disease and the Environment." (Robin Press, Lesotho 1981).

10 National Power Corporation, "Environmental Impact Statement of Naga Gas Turbine Power Project." (1989) National Power Corporation (Philippines). (unpublished).

11 V T Covello, and R S Frey, "Technology-based environmental health risks in developing nations." *Tech Forecast Soc Change*. 1990, 37:159–179.

12 J LaDou, "The export of industrial hazards to developing countries." in-*Occupational Health in Developing Countries, Ed. J Jeyaratnam*. (Oxford University Press, Oxford 1992).

13 A Mutere, "Domestic air pollution in rural Kenya." *Boiling Point – Intermediate Technology Group*. 1991, April:23–27.

14 K R Smith, "The Health Effects of Biomass Smoke: A Brief Survey of Current Knowledge." (1991) Environment and Policy Institute, Hawaii.

15 K R Smith, "Biofuels, Air Pollution and Health: A Global Review." (Plenum Press, New York 1987).

16 Intermediate Technology Development Group, "Smoke Pollution." *Boiling Point*. 1991, ?:24

17 A B Mutere, "Third Report on Tests of the Estimation of Polycyclic Aromatic Hydrocarbos (PAHs), Total Suspended Particulate (TSP) Emissions and Carbon Monoxide (CO) from Traditional and Improved Woodburning Stoves in Kiambu, Kenya, East Africa." (15 August 1990) Deutsche Gesellschaft fur Technische Zusammenarbeit.

18 J A Lee, "The Environment, Public Health and Human Ecology: Considerations for Economic Development." (John Hopkins University Press, Baltimore 1985).

19 National Power Corporation, "Environmental Impact Statement of Bacon-Manito Geothermal Project Unit 1." (1987) National Power Corporation (Philippines). (unpublished).

20 L R Anspaugh, "Health Impacts of Geothermal Energy: Extended Synopses of International Symposium on Health Impacts of Different Sources of Energy." (World Health Organization/UNEP/IAEA, Tennessee 1981).

21 J C Bhatia, "The Narmada Valley Project." in-*Health Implications of Public Policy, Ed. B Ghosh*. (Indian Institute of Management, Bangalore 1991).

22 S C Tewari, N C Appavoo, T R Mani, R Reuben, Ramadas V, and J Hiriyan, "Epidemiological aspects of persistant malaria on the river Thenpenni (Tamil Nadu)." *Indian J Med Res*. 1984, 80:1–10.

23 C L Ripert, and C P Raccurt, "The impact of small dams on parasitic diseases in Cameroon." *Parasit Today.* 1987, 3:9:287–298.

24 J M Hunter, L Rey, and D Scott, "Man-made lakes and man-made diseases; towards a policy resolution." *Soc Sci Med.* 1982, 16:1127–1145.

25 Md S Wyesundera, "Malaria outbreaks in new foci in Sri Lanka." *Parasit Today.* 1988, 4:5:147–150.

26 R W Ashford, and M C Thomson, "Visceral leishmaniasis in Sudan. A delayed development disaster?" *Ann Trop Med Parasit.* 1991, 85:5:571–572.

27 B C E Egboka, G I Nwankwor, I P Orajaka, and A O Ejiofor, "Principles and problems of environmental pollution of groundwater resources with case examples from developing countries." *Environ Hlth Perspect.* 1989, 83:39–68.

28 G Le Moigne, S Barghouti, and H Plusquellec Ed., "Dam Safety and the Environment." *World Bank Technical Paper Number 115.* (The World Bank, Washington 1989).

29 S D Helgersen, and S Milham Jr, "Farm workers electrocuted when irrigation pipes contact powerlines." *Public Health Rep.* 1985, 100:3:325–328.

chapter 6

AGRICULTURAL HEALTH HAZARDS AND THE PROJECT STAGE AT WHICH SAFEGUARDS MAY BE REQUIRED

Project stage	Health hazard	Examples and causes
Location	Communicable Disease	Contact with disease foci
	Malnutrition	Loss of subsistence crops
Planning and Design	Communicable Disease	Proliferation of vectors associated with specific crops, labourers' housing, sanitation and water supply
	Non-Communicable Disease	Agrochemical poisoning
	Malnutrition	Loss of common property resources, change of crop
	Injury	Inadequate safety measures associated with crop
Operation	Communicable Disease	Proliferation of vectors associated with specific crops, labourers' housing, sanitation and water supply
	Non-Communicable Disease	Agrochemical poisoning, toxic algal blooms
	Malnutrition	Loss of food crops, displacement of labour, changes in household entitlements, increasing workload
	Injury	Poor occupational safety, mechanization, noise

Lipton and de Kadt[1] extensively review agriculture-health linkages, identifying four components of agriculture in which health linkages can occur:

◆ Inputs, such as land, water (see *Irrigation, chapter 7*), agro-chemicals, draught power and labour;

◆ Technologies (hydraulic, mechanical, biological and post-harvest);

◆ Structures of work and ownership (including assets, laws and customs);

◆ Outputs (such as choice of crop).

Where the population is largely rural, agricultural projects are major determinants of food intake, food requirements for work, and some infectious diseases. Children's health is particularly affected by the interaction of malnutrition and infection. What children eat is partly determined by agricultural development. There is also feedback of health into agriculture. Healthier farmers and workers may be more productive and more careful, more able to risk experiments with new crops, and less likely to migrate to towns.

Many health hazards arise from contact with agricultural produce, domestic animals, animal excreta, animal products and human excreta used as fertilizer. See also *Livestock, chapter 10 and Manufacture and Trade, chapter 12, Agricultural Processing Industries.*

1   AGRICULTURAL LABOUR

Landless agricultural labourers are a vulnerable group because of low and unstable wages and low levels of employment[1]. They may, for example, be unable to purchase sufficient food during the slack season. The high energy requirements of manual labour may exceed the energy levels of food intake. Farm workers are exposed to new hazards of agro-chemical poisoning and machinery besides traditional health hazards of bites and stings, dehydration and back injury. The shift in Asia from increasing draught power to tractors usually displaces labour without increasing output. This shift is often encouraged by providing credit or by subsidising fuel and tractors.

EXAMPLES

◆ Traditional agricultural hazards accounted for 5% of time spent off work by casual rural labourers in India during 1977–8[1].

◆ During periods of food shortage young farm workers in India, Ethiopia and Bangladesh are poisoned by consuming the grass pea[2,3,4].

Women gain mixed benefits from agricultural labour. The extra income may provide extra food but the type of work may be incompatible with child care.

As men move out of the fields and into the cash economy, women's role in subsistence production has increased. The replacement of subsistence crops by cash crops often has a direct effect on women. Where a woman's workload is increased there may be reduced time to care for her family or attend at health clinics. This increases children's exposure to diseases, malnutrition and injuries. Mechanization alters the division of labour. Tractors and irrigation bring larger areas under cultivation, giving women increased land to weed. Intensive sugar cane production requires more weeding on the same unit of land.

EXAMPLES

◆ In the foothills of the Indian Himalayas women perform 75% of the agricultural work and 90% of the cattle care[5].

◆ In Gujerat, poor women agricultural labourers take time off from paid daily work in the fields to deliver their children. They become indebted to the extent of the number of days' wages they have lost. The high interest rate charged further impoverishes the household[6].

1.1 COMMUNICABLE DISEASE

Commercial agriculture often employs seasonal migrant labour who may be more susceptible to communicable diseases such as malaria[7]. *See also Cross-Cutting Issues, chapter 2, Labour Mobility and below, Plantation Agriculture.*

EXAMPLE

◆ A study in Thailand contrasted malaria in sugar cane plantation owners with malaria in migrant labourers from a non-malarious region. The migrants knew less about transmission, had less access to mosquito nets, were less likely to take anti-malarial drugs and had a higher malaria prevalence[7.]

Women may grow or make products for sale but have no access to markets. They may be required to trade sexual favours to obtain market access (such as transport from truck drivers), credit, raw materials, or wage labour. This enhances the transmission of STDs into uninfected populations.

Latrines are rarely incorporated in farm plans. Open defecation leads to disease transmission. Cheap, shallow pit latrines are often all that is required.

2   CHOICE OF CROP

2.1   COMMUNICABLE DISEASE

Rice cultivation is nearly always associated with an increase in malaria. However, in sub-saharan Africa malaria transmission is sometimes already at saturation level so that increases in vector breeding may have no effect. In some areas of West Africa the irrigated fields are colonised by a mosquito sub-species that appears to be a poor malaria vector[8]. There is a succession of different mosquito species in rice fields as sun-loving species are replaced by shade-loving species when the rice grows. New high yielding varieties (HYVs) produce less shade and may alter this succession. On the other hand the large amounts of fertilizer and pesticide used with HYVs may deter certain malaria vectors. They may also adversely affect existing aquatic food chains and soil microorganisms including mosquito (larvae) predators.

EXAMPLES

◆ The malaria vector *An. culicifacies* used to be very common in Indian rice fields but is now much reduced in some areas, possibly due to the introduction of new rice varieties[9].

◆ At Bura, in Kenya, there was initially a plan to cultivate rice. This was changed to cotton cultivation when it was recognised that uncontrollable malaria transmission could result[10].

2.2   NON-COMMUNICABLE DISEASE

There are special occupational hazards associated with particular crops[11,12]. The agricultural tasks associated with these crops may tend to be gender specific. For example, women may be employed for tea and tobacco picking. Teapickers are exposed to high levels of pesticides used in tea growing. *See also Manufacture and Trade, chapter 12, Agricultural Processing Industries.*

Certain varieties of crops, such as cassava, contain toxins. Promotion of these varieties may be associated with a real risk of poisoning among consumers. Production and consumption of the grass-pea is increasing in India, Ethiopia and Bangladesh. Over-consumption of improperly cooked grass-pea leads to lathyrism, a neurotoxic disorder, common in young men[3].

EXAMPLES

◆ Tobacco cultivation is very labour intensive and requires labour in short duration peaks, which disrupts employment patterns. The capital investment is often provided by the company, the farmers become indebted and may lose their freedom of choice[13]. Tobacco also requires large quantities of fertilizers, pesticides and herbicides that are largely unmonitored and penetrate water ways and food chains posing a threat to human health and may cause problems of pesticide resistant disease vectors[14].

◆ 'Green syndrome' is an occupational health hazard associated with picking and curing tobacco leaves[11].

◆ Rice planters suffer keratitis as an occupational eye disease[15].

◆ The grass-pea is especially tolerant to drought, poor soils and pest attack. It can be intercropped and is useful for nitrogen fixation. These characteristics make it attractive to poor peasants, especially during times of stress. In an Ethiopian study, consumers were aware of its toxic potential but found it preferable to starvation[3].

2.3 MALNUTRITION

Food security means physical and economic access to food for all people at all times. Lack of food security is associated with poor nutritional status, particularly in young children[16,17]. The malnourished child is more susceptible to communicable disease. Food insecurity is a concrete manifestation of poverty that may be more meaningful than income levels.

The combination of low intensity of infection with many different species of parasites in conjunction with inadequate diet probably has a major nutritional effect on children. In rural Tanzania malnutrition in school children was closely correlated with multiple infections with *Ascaris*, hookworm and *Schistosoma*[18].

Changes in household food security and nutritional status can occur, for example when projects affect: food production, food availability, purchasing power, feeding practices, prevalence of infections, and workload.

EXAMPLES

◆ A Kenyan study assessed the link between malnutrition and production of a specific cash crop. Children of families who grew the crop were compared with children living in the same ecological zone but not involved in cash cropping. Sugar production was significantly associated with malnutrition as was a switch from traditional weaning foods to commercialized food substitutes. Smallholder tea growing in Kericho district was associated with a serious reduction in home-produced food. Results from cotton and pyrethrum growers were neutral. Other tea and coffee results were inconsistent[19].

◆ A positive change in nutritional status was observed on a paddy rice development scheme in Sri Lanka. It was noted that rice was a traditional crop which had cultural and nutritional importance in the community. The scheme provided a surplus of the traditional crop which could be stored, against seasonal fluctuations, or sold[20].

Transitory and chronic forms of food insecurity are recognised. Transitory food insecurity can be associated with seasonal shortages or, for example, a shift from subsistence to cash crops. Changes from subsistence to cash crops may reduce the availability of subsistence food crops within the home. Income may be insufficient to buy food in local markets. The price of market food may rise. Cash may be controlled by male members of the household who do not use it for the benefit of the elderly, women and children.

Crop development programmes may neglect staple root crops and coarse grains in favour of high protein or fine grain export crops. They may reduce the income or security of vulnerable groups, reduce the production of foods for home consumption or increase the price of purchased foods.

Crops with a high value, high yield and high protein content may represent a health hazard to poor farmers by paradoxically increasing malnutrition[1]. Such crops may not meet the needs of poor people for the following reasons.

The poor need:
◆ Subsistence rather than cash crops.
◆ Extra energy rather than extra protein.
◆ Reliable yields rather than high yields.
◆ Stable market demand rather than extreme price fluctuations.
◆ Varieties that are resistant to drought and disease, easy to store and require limited labour.

High yielding varieties may be deficient in micronutrients such as iron, vitamin A, iodine or niacin.

Promotion of export crops (often associated with structural adjustment programmes) may adversely affect production of food crops through competition for productive resources, but the available evidence is mixed[21]. The effect of cash crop production on income and nutrition is mixed[22]. Change from subsistence to cash cropping is usually accompanied by a reduction in crop diversity. The simplification of traditional diets can lead to nutritional imbalance and increasing malnutrition[23].

EXAMPLES

◆ In 1991 tobacco was the most widely grown non-food crop in 120 countries, it usurped the place of food crops which could feed an estimated 10 to 20 million people[14].

◆ One acre of forest is required to cure one acre of tobacco, resulting in an estimated 7 million acres of land deforested each year. This leads to problems of global warming, soil erosion and tropical flooding which decrease the capacity of the land to be used for food production and contributes to food insecurity[14,24].

On the other hand, there are crops such as tea, where the nature of the land and the market ensures a more stable employment from an export than from a staple crop. In Africa, it has been suggested that change to modern varieties of crops may be less harmful than no change at all[1].

The poor usually obtain their sustenance more from vegetable than animal foods. Animal development projects may divert land from producing staple crops and reduce the food supply of the poor.

2.4   INJURY

The cultivation, harvesting and processing of crops may expose workers to a range of injury hazards that are crop specific. For example teapickers are exposed to injuries and falls associated with steep slopes, insect and snake bites.

See also Manufacture and Trade, chapter 12, Agricultural Processing Industries.

3   AGRO-CHEMICALS

3.1   COMMUNICABLE DISEASE

Field breeding mosquitoes are one of the non-target organisms affected by pesticide use. Cross-resistant strains are selected which are difficult for the public health sector to control. The prevalence of malaria may then increase. This problem could be reduced if some categories of insecticide were reserved for public health use, as has happened in Sri Lanka. However, such schemes are difficult to regulate and do not overcome problems of cross-resistance.

3.2   NON-COMMUNICABLE DISEASE

See also Manufacture and Trade, chapter 12, Agricultural Processing Industries.

Poisoning can cause both non-communicable disease and injury. For convenience we discuss all forms of agro-chemical poisoning in this section.

The level of risk to exposure to chemicals is usually higher in intensive farming and horticulture than in traditional farming[25].

It has been estimated that, in developing countries, 3 million people suffer from single short-term exposure to chemicals (including suicide or attempted suicide) with 220,000 deaths. Fatality rates vary from 1% to 9% in cases presenting for treatment according to the level of service available. Over 700,000 people a year are thought to suffer from the chronic effects of long-term exposure. The scale and nature of such effects may be underestimated. The symptoms of pesticide poisoning may be incorrectly ascribed to other causes. The main factors contributing to mortality are believed to include environmental contamination, unintentional exposure during work, errors in preparation, failure to use protective clothing and suicide[25].

Unintentional acute or chronic pesticide poisoning is an occupational hazard of farm workers. It is a growing and serious problem, but poorly documented[26,27,28]. Some 50 million people have regular contact with pesticides and 500 million have less regular contact. The latter category may be particularly at risk because they will usually be less well informed of the hazards. A disturbing trend is the unrestricted use of highly toxic organophosphates such as methyl parathion and monocrotophos. Cases of pesticide poisoning are often misdiagnosed.

Acute pesticide poisoning has received more attention than the chronic effects of poisoning. Recently circumstantial evidence has been published of increased adult male mortality in intensive rice production systems in North Luzon, Philippines. Detailed studies at the International Rice Research Institute (IRRI), in the Philippines, are underway which tend to confirm the evidence of chronic poisoning. The IRRI reiterate the need for integrated pest management and have developed more pest resistant strains of rice. It is possible and practical to monitor pesticide exposure by routine medical examination.

Many older and more toxic pesticides are still available in stores and market places. Their cheap price makes them attractive to smaller farmers who may thereby circumvent donor policy. This may be of particular concern in smallholder agricultural development.

There may be over one million cases of unintentional pesticide poisoning per year[29]. Low levels of literacy and education in rural communities with poor access to training increase the risk of pesticide poisoning. Pesticide is often applied by itinerant, unskilled, unsupervised operators. It is still common to observe storing, mixing, application and disposal without adequate safety precautions. Lack of proper supervision also increases the risk of pesticide poisoning. Protective clothing of the type used in northern countries is too expensive and unsuitable for hot countries. The Pesticide Management Section of the Natural Resources Institute advocates the use of lightweight cotton overalls that are frequently washed as well as gloves and disposable face masks. Poor access to water and soap for decontamination is a further risk factor. Operatives frequently eat and smoke during spraying operations. Aerial spraying of insecticides often contaminates operatives, casual bystanders and local fauna, resulting in serious levels of exposure especially to organophosphorous type compounds. Reports of both domestic animals and human deaths have been seen in South Africa, Cuba and West Africa[30].

A recent study from the Philippines suggested that the cost of ill-health from pesticide exposure may be greater than the value of the extra crop produced[28].

EXAMPLE

◆ A study in Malaysia suggested that 92% of agricultural workers used pesticides. Of these some 7% had been poisoned in one year. Hospital admissions for pesticide poisoning were composed of 14–32% occupational poisonings and an equal number of non-occupational unintentional poisoning. In a study in Sri Lanka some 70% of unintentional poisonings were due to occupational exposure. In Latin America some 10–30% of agricultural workers showed evidence of pesticide poisoning in certain selected groups. Studies of intense rice cultivation in the Philippines has attributed both mortality and morbidity to chronic pesticide exposure[31].

Unintentional mass poisoning with agro-chemicals is more dramatic but rarer. It occurs when people consume treated grains or contaminated stored produce. In Iraq some 6,350 people were admitted to hospital and more than

459 died, after eating bread prepared from cereals treated with methyl mercury fungicide[32]. Parathion has been responsible for mass poisoning in India, Egypt, Colombia and Mexico. Hexachlorohexane treated grain caused 3000 cases of poisoning in Turkey.

Unintentional poisoning due to the use of pesticide/chemical containers as cooking utensils, for water storage and collection is a major hazard. Such empty containers are often sold in the markets to poor people. Poor labelling may cause people to ingest insecticide by mistake.

EXAMPLE

◆ Insecticide taken as sugar in Dar es Salaam in 1974 caused 28 hospitalised deaths[30].

Pesticide residues in locally grown vegetables are frequently far in excess of the acceptable limits. Green leafy vegetables are especially at risk[33]. Many species of wild food, including fish, molluscs, crustacea, insects and vegetables, are harvested among cultivated crops. Such foods are especially important for the landless poor and for children. Pesticides may either remove or contaminate such foods. Residues and propellants can deoxygenate waters causing large scale fauna depletion and food loss.

Exported foods, including fruits and meats, are rejected at the port of entry in the UK, if they contain higher residues of pesticide than locally grown produce.

EXAMPLE

◆ A locust outbreak in 1989 in Lesotho was controlled by use of un-labelled, un-named insecticides by untrained personnel supplied with ULV sprays, masks and gloves. The spraying killed locusts and many birds. Human effects were not reported[30].

The global use of nitrogen fertilizers has increased exponentially since the second world war. Much of the recent increase has been in developing countries and in support of HYV cereals. Most fertilizer is lost to surface and ground-water, finding its way into drinking supplies. There is a documented risk that nitrates may be converted to nitrites in the human gut through the action of bacteria[34]. Nitrites bind to haemoglobin, impairing the transport of oxygen. The potential risk is greatest in bottle-fed infants and gives rise to the blue-baby syndrome. At present the condition is rare but there is concern for its future increase.

Pesticides, particularly herbicides, have been found in drinking water. High levels of chlorinated hydrocarbon pesticides have been reported in water in Colombia, Malaysia, Thailand and Tanzania[25].

Nitrogen and phosphate contamination of the drinking water reservoirs can stimulate production of harmful toxins by blue green algae[35]. Toxic algal blooms associated with agricultural run-off can cause dermatitis and gastro-intestinal disease. Livestock may be killed.

EXAMPLE

◆ 6,000 personnel at Clark US Air Base, Philippines, suffered diarrhoea during summer epidemics of cyanobacteria in drinking water[36].

---

4 PLANTATION AGRICULTURE

See also Forestry, chapter 9, and Cross-Cutting Issues, chapter 2, Labour Mobility.

Plantations are frequently developed to support export crop production. They have many similarities that are independent of region or government[37]. They employ labour living in enclaves that may be physically or culturally isolated from other communities. There is considerable information concerning the harsh social conditions experienced by the plantation workforce and the increasing labour militancy that this can provoke[38]. Contributing factors to poor health include: seasonal unemployment, mechanization, poor housing, inadequate diets and lack of access to health care and education. Health care facilities may be restricted to skilled workers; women, children and contract workers may be excluded. Health care facilities may not be planned for ease of access by workers, wages may be lost if they attend during working hours. This can affect the uptake of immunization and antenatal services. Child mortality and morbidity rates are frequently higher on plantations. Health services tend to be entirely curative with little attempt at sanitation, environmental protection or vector control.

On the other hand, plantation managers can deliver health care to an easily identified workforce. Plantation vehicles may be used as transport to remote health centres which would otherwise be inaccessible.

Plantations may dispossess subsistence farmers of their land and make them landless labourers. Non-permanent labour often has the poorest housing, lacking environmental health provision. On average, 80% of the agricultural worker's wage is spent on food. High-priced commercial foods may be consumed as a result of poor access to peasant markets. Food security is poor where labourers have no rights to gardens of their own.

EXAMPLES

◆ When the tea estates in Sri Lanka were nationalised during the mid-70's, the poor health and welfare conditions of the labourers received public attention. Chronic malnutrition and infant mortality rates were twice the rural average. Child labour was common; education facilities were minimal. Water supplies were inadequate. State ownership, uniform health policies and donor assistance have since led to a substantial improvement[37].

◆ In Zimbabwe, during 1981, the rates of acute and chronic malnutrition were higher among commercial farm labour communities than in any other sector, including the communal areas[37].

◆ There was widespread malnutrition on Malaysian rubber estates during the 1970's. Worm infestation, leptospirosis antibodies and snake bite were common. However, water supply and sanitation were good. Houses were well-built but overcrowded[15].

◆ An 8,000 ha palm oil estate was developed on Mindanao, Philippines. The land was designated and already occupied by 2,000 farmers who were violently forced off their land. Human rights abuses were confirmed in 1983. A community of independent farmers producing food for local consumption was transformed into wage labour producing industrial raw material for export necessitating child labour for family units to survive[39]. This could be expected to produce food insecurity and health problems associated with child labour.

4.1 COMMUNICABLE DISEASE

Communicable diseases on plantations may be exacerbated by poor conditions or by the importation of low paid labour from endemic regions[40].

Tree crop plantations often provide habitats for shade-loving vectors and the animal reservoirs of certain parasitic infections[41]. The associated diseases may be an occupational hazard of plantation workers or may be more widely distributed among their dependants. For example, rubber plantation workers contract malaria as an occupational hazard because they cut the trees during the hours of darkness. Plantation workers in the riverine areas where the black fly *Simulium damnosum* is present can contract onchocerciasis causing considerable morbidity[42].

EXAMPLES

◆ In Swaziland, lowland sugar estate development followed successful malaria control. Swazi men avoided employment on the estates because of the poor living and working conditions. The estate managers chose to employ migrant Mozambique labour, providing a new malaria reservoir, despite health sector warnings. Swazi women and children were also employed as casual labourers. There was a resurgence of malaria that could not be attributed to pesticide resistance[40].

◆ Sub-periodic Brugian filariasis is transmitted by *Mansonia* mosquitoes in Malaysian rubber estates. The estates are surrounded by swamp forest inhabited by monkeys which are heavily infected with the parasite. The monkeys are frequently found in the estates near to human habitation. The infection is present in estate workers and their dependents[41].

Epidemics of mucocutaneous leishmaniasis are reported from coffee plantations in the Andes. The sandfly vector rests and feeds in the shade of the coffee bushes[43].

4.2   MALNUTRITION

New plantations are established in support of resettlement schemes in programmes of smallholder agricultural development. The smallholders are often switched from subsistence to cash crops. Success may depend on the availability of food gardens. Nutritional problems are common.

EXAMPLES

◆ Ten thousand smallholders were settled on an oil palm scheme in Papua New Guinea. Each smallholder established food gardens under the growing oil palms. These produced a substantial surplus which was traded in the local markets for other foods such as fish. There was considerable entrepreneurial activity. When the oil palm canopy closed the food intercropping would no longer be possible. It was recommended that blocks be permanently set aside for food gardens so that food production could continue[44,45].

◆ By contrast, in a different Papua New Guinean study an increase in underweight children was noted two years after the commencement of a rubber resettlement project. The effect was attributed to transitional malnutrition as it takes several years to earn returns from a rubber plantation[19].

---

5   MECHANIZATION AND AGRICULTURE

5.1   COMMUNICABLE DISEASE

Reduction of livestock associated with a switch to mechanized agriculture has been associated with malaria outbreaks when the vector switches to feeding on a human host[46]. Mechanization may increase the number of rice crops that can be grown during the year and extend the malaria transmission season[8].

Increased mechanization may reduce the transmission of vector-borne diseases. Larger more fertile fields and improved drains reduce breeding sites. Schistosomiasis may decrease as a result of decreased water contact[25].

5.2   MALNUTRITION

Agricultural mechanization may increase the demand on women for low-productivity and physically demanding work. At the same time, it may reduce the male workload and increase male control over the processes. Even where labour saving technologies have been introduced for traditional female work, they have sometimes been handed over to male control[47]. This decreases the income of women and their food security, reinforces their position as unable to manage machines, places strains on their nutritional resources and reduces the time and energy available for child care and food preparation.

EXAMPLE

◆   Introduction of a mechanical rice husker in Bangladesh, controlled by men, removed one of the few income generating options open to poor rural women[48].

Reducing labour intensive occupations and displacing labourers can lead to reduced food security for vulnerable groups.

Cost of tractor hire/use is so great in smaller fields that it drastically reduces family income from land especially in regions of high unemployment and results in food scarcity as in the case of most of Lesotho[30].

5.3   INJURY

The frequency of traumatic injuries is likely to change with increased mechanization. For example, very high rates of injury are reported among sugar cane workers. The injuries occur from the use of heavy machetes. Ulcerous sores are also caused by minute hairs on the sugar cane stalk[49].

Tractors are well known as an important cause of agricultural injuries. They are unstable because of their need for high ground clearance. Adults and children living in rural areas of developing countries often have very little appreciation of the dangers associated with these vehicles.

EXAMPLES

◆ In Uganda, although only 21% of the employed persons were engaged in agriculture in 1987, they accounted for 33% of all occupational injuries[50].

◆ In the UK most farm injuries are associated with machinery[33].

◆ An extensive study in India identified the causes of agricultural injuries. Spades and sickles were most commonly implicated; severe injuries were associated with the use of poorly designed fodder cutters and threshers. 45% of fodder cutter injuries were sustained by children[51].

The high noise levels associated with agricultural machinery may induce hearing loss as well as stress and behavioural problems[25].

6 REFERENCES

1 M Lipton, and E de Kadt, "Agriculture-Health Linkages." *Offset Publication No. 104*, (World Health Organization, Geneva 1988).

2 M P Dwivedi, and B G Prasad, "An epidemiological study of lathyrism in the district of Rewa, Madhya Pradesh." *Indian J Med Res.* 1964, 52:81–116.

3 R T Haimanot, Y Kidane, E Wuhib, A Kalissa, T Alemu, Z A Zein, and P S Spencer, "Lathyrism in rural northwest Ethiopia: a highly prevalent neurotoxic disorder." *Intern J Epid.* 1990, 19:3:664–672.

4 V S Palmer, A K Kaul, and P S Spencer, "International network for the improvement of Lathyrus sativus and the eradication of lathyrism (INILSEL): a TWMRF initiative." in-*Grass-pea: Threat and Promise, Ed. P S Spencer.* (Third World Medical Research Foundation, New York 1989).

5 M Sarin, "Himachali Women – A Situational Analysis." (December 1989) UNICEF.

6 E Bhatt, M Chatterjee, and J Price, "Towards Maternal Protection." (1986) Self Employed Women's Association, Ahmedabad. (unpublished).

7 W Kanjanapan, "Health effects of labour mobility: A study of malaria in Kanchanaburi Province, Thailand." *Southeast Asian J Trop Med Public Health.* 1983, 14:1:54–57.

8 M W Service, "The importance of ecological studies on malaria vectors." *Bull Soc Vector Ecol.* 1989, 14:1:26–38.

9 R Reuben, "Obstacles to malaria control in India – the human factor." in-*Demography and Vector-Borne Diseases, Ed. M W Service.* (CRC Press, Florida 1989).

10 D H Smith, Personal communication.

11 S K Ghosh, J R Parikh, V N Gokani, S K Kashyap, and S K Chatterjee, "Studies on occupational health problems during agricultural operation of Indian tobacco workers. A preliminary survey report." *J Occup Med.* 1979, 21:1:45–47.

12 Nag Anjali, "Occupational Health Hazards for Women in India." (1986) National Institute of Occupational Health, Women's Cell, Ahmedabad, Gujerat, India.

13 K Brott, "Tobacco smoking in Papua New Guinea." *Papua New Guinea Med J.* 1981, 24:4:229–236.

14 M Barry, "The influence of the US tobacco industry on the health, economy and environment of developing countries." *N Eng J Med.* 1991, 324:13:917–920.

15 Lim Heng Huat, "Health problems of agricultural workers in Malaysia." *Trop Geogr Med.* 1983, 35:83–89.

16 P R Payne, "Measuring malnutrition." *IDS Bull.* 1990, 21:3:14–30.

17 P J Dearden, and E M Cassidy, "Food security: an ODA view." *IDS Bull.* 1990, 21:3:81–83.

18 R H Meakins, P S E G Harland, and F Carswell, "A preliminary survey of malnutrition and helminthiasis among school children in one mountain and one lowland ujamaa village in Northern Tanzania." *Trans R Soc Trop Med Hyg.* 1981, 75:5:731–735.

19 C M Fillmore, and M A Hussain, "Agriculture and anthropometry: assessing the nutritional impact." *Food & Nutr.* 1984, 10:2:2–14.

20 G Holmboe-Ottesen, M Wandel, and A Oshaug, "Nutritional evaluation of an agricultural development project in southern Sri Lanka." *Food & Nutr.* 1989, 11:3:47–56.

21 D E C Cooper Weil, A P Alicbusan, J F Wilson, M R Reich, and D J Bradley, "The Impact of Development Policies on Health: A Review of the Literature." (World Health Organization, Geneva 1990).

22 R Longhurst, "Cash crops, household food security and nutrition." *IDS Bull.* 1988, 19:2:28–36.

23 P Fleuret, and A Fleuret, "Nutrition, consumption, and agricultural change." *Hum Org.* 1980, 39:3:250–260.

24 K R Stebbins, "Transnational tobacco companies and health in underdeveloped countries: recommendations for avoiding a smoking epidemic." *Soc Sci Med.* 1990, 30:2:227–235.

25 World Health Organization Commission on Health and Environment, "Our Planet, Our Health." (World Health Organization, Geneva 1992).

26 M E Loevinsohn, "Insecticide use and increased mortality in rural Central Luzon, Philippines." *The Lancet.* 1987, 332:8546:1359–1362.

27 J A McCracken, and G R Conway, "Pesticide Hazards in the Third World: New Evidence From the Philippines." (September 1987) International Institute for Environment and Development. SA1.

28 P L Pingali, and C Marquez, "Health costs of long term pesticide exposure in the Philippines – a medical and economic analysis." (1990) Annual General Meeting of the American Agricultural Economics Association. vol. 90–04. Vancouver BC, Canada. Social Science Division, International Rice Research Institute, Manila, Philippines.

29 World Health Organization, "Informal Consultation on Planning for the

Prevention of Pesticide Poisoning." (1986) World Health Organization. VBC/86.926.

30 R H Meakins, Personal communication.

31 World Health Organization/United Nations Environment Programme Working Group on Public Health Impact of Pesticides Used in Agriculture, "Public Health Impact of Pesticides Used in Agriculture." (World Health Organization and United Nations Environment Programme, Geneva 1990).

32 D Bull, "A Growing Problem: Pesticides and the Thirld World Poor." (Oxfam, Oxford 1982).

33 G R Conway, and J N Pretty, "Unwelcome Harvest: Agriculture and Pollution." (Earthscan Publications, London 1991).

34 G R Conway, and J N Pretty, "Fertilizer risks in the developing countries." *Nature.* 1988, 334:6179:207–208.

35 P C Turner, A J Gammie, K Hollinrake, and G A Codd, "Pneumonia associated with cyanobacteria." *Brit Med J.* 1990, 300:1440–1441.

36 P R Hunter, "Human illness associated with freshwater cyanobacteria (blue-green algae)." *Public Health Laboratory Service Microbiol Dig.* 1991, 8:3:96–100.

37 R Laing, "Health and Health Services for Plantation Workers: Four Case Studies." *EPC Publication No.10,* (Evaluation and Planning Centre for Health Care, London School of Hygiene and Tropical Medicine, London 1986).

38 R Loewenson, "Challenges to health in plantation economies: recent trends." *Hlth Policy Plng.* 1989, 4:4:334–342.

39 P Lee-Wright, "Child Slaves." (Earthscan, London 1990).

40 R M Packard, "Agricultural development, migrant labour and the resurgence of malaria in Swaziland." *Soc Sci Med.* 1986, 22:8:861–867.

41 J W Mak, W H Cheong, P K F Yen, P K C Lin, and W C Chan, "Studies on the epidemiology of sub-periodic *Brugia malayi* in Malaysia: problems in its control." *Acta Tropica.* 1982, 39:237–245.

42 I G Thomson, "Onchocerciasis oil palm estate." *Trans R Soc Trop Med Hyg.* 1971, 65:4:484–489.

43 A Warburg, J Montoya-Lerma, C Jaramillo, A L Cruz-Ruiz, and K Ostrovska, "Leishmaniasis vector potential of *Lutzomyia* spp. in Columbian coffee plantations." *Med Vet Ent.* 1991, 5:9–16.

44 C Benjamin, "Some food market influences of a large-scale small-holder development in the West New Britain area of Papua New Guimea." *Papua New Guinea Journal of Agriculture, Forestry and Fisheries.* 1985, 33:3–4:133–141.

45 C Benjamin, and I Wapi, "Subsistence gardening on the Hoskins Oil Palm Scheme." (1980) R M Bourke and V Kesavan Ed., Second Papua New Guinea Food Crops Conference. vol. 1. Goroka Teachers'College, Goroka, Papua New Guinea. Department of Primary Industry, Port Moresby, Papua New Guinea.

46 S K Ault, "Effect of demographic patterns, social structure, and human behaviour on malaria." in-*Demography and Vector-Borne Diseases, Ed. M W Service.* (CRC Press, Florida 1989).

47 B Rogers, "The Domestication of Women." (Tavistock Publications Ltd, London 1981).

48 M Greeley, "Postharvest Losses, Technology and Employment: The Case of Rice in Bangladesh." *Westview Special Studies in Social, Political and Economic Development,* (Westview Press, Boulder Colorado, USA 1987).

49 H Phool Chund, "Health and safety in agriculture: the sugarcane industry." *African Newsletter on Occupational Health and Safety*. 1991, 1:3:83–85.
50 D K Sekimpi, "Occupational health services for agricultural workers." in- *Occupational Health in Developing Countries, Ed. J Jeyaratnam*. (Oxford University Press, Oxford 1992).
51 D Mohan, I Qadeer, R Patel, M Varghese, S J Shah, H Kumar, L S Chahar, M Guar, and A Kumar, "Grains of Blood: Prevention and Control of Farm Injuries in India." (13 February 1992) WHO Collaborating Centre for Research and Training in Safety Technology, Centre for Biomedical Engineering, Indian Institute of Technology, Delhi.

chapter 7

IRRIGATION

IRRIGATION HEALTH HAZARDS AND THE PROJECT STAGE AT WHICH SAFEGUARDS MAY BE REQUIRED

Project stage	Health hazard	Examples and causes
Location	Communicable Disease	Contact with disease foci, domestic water supply contamination
	Malnutrition	Loss of subsistence crops
	Injury	Floods, drowning
Planning and Design	Communicable Disease	Sanitary waste disposal
	Non-Communicable Disease	Water pollution
Construction	Communicable Disease	Poor sanitation, water supply and food hygiene, STDs, exposure to vectors
	Non-Communicable Disease	Inadequate occupational safety measures
	Injury	Inadequate occupational safety measures
Operation	Communicable Disease	Creation of vector habitats, water and vector exposure, wastewater re-use in agriculture
	Non-Communicable Disease	Leachates in drinking water, mineral salt uptake by food crops

1   COMMUNICABLE DISEASE

The problems of vector-borne disease associated with irrigation and dams have received considerable attention for many years[1,2,3,4,5]. Unfortunately, this has not yet been accompanied by significant changes in policy, planning or operational procedures. *See also Energy, chapter 5, Hydropower.*

EXAMPLE

◆ A study has indicated that the incidence of malaria, filariasis, cholera, gastroenteritis and goitre are likely to increase as a result of the Narmada Sagar Dam in India[6].

Irrigation projects cause profound ecological change that often encourages mosquito breeding. No one knows how much malaria is associated with irrigation, but many of the world's most efficient malaria vectors breed in or around rice fields. Unfortunately, malaria almost invariably increases as a result of surface irrigation.

General environmental changes brought about by irrigation practices which may have effects on health are:-

◆ Simplification of the habitat;

◆ Increase in the area of surface water;

◆ A rise in the water table;

◆ Changes in the rate of water flow;

◆ A modification of the microclimate;

◆ Urban development[7].

EXAMPLES

◆ People living on the Ahero rice irrigation scheme, Kenya, are bitten up to 70 times more by malaria vectors, compared with those living outside the scheme[8].

◆ In Afghanistan, the Kunduz valley was developed during the 1960's for the cultivation of rice, cotton and vegetables. The rice fields and irrigation canal overflows created ideal mosquito breeding sites and *vivax* malaria incidence increased from 5% to 20%. Malaria incidence is now highest in irrigated rice field areas, where most of the population live[9].

◆ In the 1000km² rice growing area of the Ruzizi valley, Burundi, dry season malaria is more common than in neighbouring cotton producing areas[10].

Irrigation of semi-arid areas lengthens the malaria transmission season.

Much malaria associated with irrigation is due to untidy practices and various simple measures could be taken to prevent outbreaks. Efficient water use is often the key to reduced vector breeding. The key to efficient water use and the maintenance of water channels lies with the division of responsibility and financing between the individual, the community, the irrigation system management and the government[11,12].

The public health importance of schistosomiasis in irrigation projects has often been emphasised. It arises as an occupational hazard of farmers, a recreational hazard of bathers and a domestic hazard, eg. fetching water, washing. The severity of the disease is a function of the intensity of infection. Intensity increases where communities are exposed to contaminated water for extended periods. Irrigation extends water contact leading to increasing intensity of infection.

EXAMPLE

◆ Traditionally the annual Nile flood was seasonal. The construction of the Upper Aswan Dam in the 1960s enabled perennial irrigation, reduced the silt load in the river and encouraged the growth of aquatic plants. The environmental changes extended the habitat for snail vectors. Farmers spent a longer time during the year in contact with water. The prevalence of *Schistosoma haematobium* in the Aswan area increased from 13% in 1937 to 32% in 1972. Following programmes of health education, chemotherapy and snail control, prevalence of *S.haematobium* in the Aswan area was reduced to 12% by 1982[13].

Migrant labour has been responsible for the importation of schistosomiasis into new irrigation schemes. Returning labourers may then transmit the disease to new areas, as happened in the Awash Valley of Ethiopia[14]. *See also Cross-Cutting Issues, chapter 2, Labour Mobility.*

There was a rapid rise in the prevalence of schistosomiasis in Ghana after the construction of the dam that created Lake Volta. The same may happen in India with the current construction of the Narmada Valley Development Project, although the parasite is currently rare in India. In many dry areas in Africa (Nigeria, Kenya, Cameroon) the development of small dams and reservoirs has increased the prevalence and intensity of infection with both schistosomiasis and dracunculiasis[15]. *See also Energy, chapter 5.*

Several acute mosquito-borne arbovirus infections are important in irrigation schemes. They are often associated with a bird or animal reservoir of infection. Japanese Encephalitis (JE) is an example.

EXAMPLE

◆ The Mahaweli rice development project in Sri Lanka provided breeding sites for the mosquito vector of JE. A separate development project encouraged pig production near the rice fields. Pigs are the reservoir hosts of the JE virus. Epidemics seriously disrupted the newly settled communities[16].

Building of dams for irrigation in areas where the black fly is present increases the transmission of onchocerciasis[17]. Other potential problems are listed in a recent WHO publication[5].

Despite the intentions of planners, communities will use irrigation water for domestic purposes, especially during the dry season. They may also defecate on the banks of canals and use the water for anal cleansing.

Well planned irrigation can complement domestic water provision, especially in the dry season.

Wastewater containing pathogens and heavy metals is increasingly being used for irrigation. Correlations between wastewater use and children's diarrhoea have been observed. The development of appropriate safety measures is of current concern[18].

EXAMPLE

◆ About 50% of the water-borne sewage produced in India is used for irrigation[19].

Withdrawing fresh water from rivers for irrigation may affect the quantity available to dilute and carry wastewater.

2   NON-COMMUNICABLE DISEASE

See also Cross-Cutting Issues, chapter 2, Resettlement.

Irrigation return water contains more salts than the original supply, due to leaching from the root zone. High levels of salts in drinking water make it unpalatable, creating downstream drinking water shortages. Increased salt levels in drinking water associated with salts and fertilizers has been regarded as a major cause of high blood pressure in regions where bore hole water is commonly used, such as Lesotho[20]. Consumption of plants grown in such water can sometimes induce crippling bone diseases[6,21].

EXAMPLE

◆ People in areas around the Nagarjuna Sagar Dam in India have suffered a high incidence in fluorosis and genu valgum (knocked knees syndrome) due to soil environmental changes[6].

---

3 INJURY

Drowning is a significant cause of injury deaths in many developing countries. Although there is little information about the precise sites of drowning (sea, lakes, rivers, ponds, wells or irrigation canals) it can be predicted that extending irrigation systems, including dams and canals, will lead to an increase in exposure to water and potentially to increase deaths from drowning. This is especially so in situations where the water mass is not protected by any fencing or covers.

4 REFERENCES

1 J M Hunter, L Rey, K Y Chu, E O Adekolu-John, and K E Mott, "Parasitic diseases in water resources development." (WHO, Geneva 1993).

2 J M V Oomen, J de Wolf, and W R Jobin, "Health and Irrigation. Incorporation of disease control measures in irrigation, a multi-faceted task in design, construction, operation – Volume 2." 2 (International Institute for Land Reclamation and Improvement, Wageningen, Netherlands 1988).

3 J M V Oomen, J de Wolf, and W R Jobin, "Health and Irrigation. Incorporation of disease control measures in irrigation, a multi-faceted task in design, construction, operation." 1 (International Institute for Land Reclamation and Improvement, Wageningen, The Netherlands 1990).

4 M Tiffen, "Guidelines for the Incorporation of Health Safeguards into Irrigation Projects Through Intersectoral Cooperation." *PEEM Guidelines, No.1*, (WHO/FAO/UNEP, 1989).

5 M H Birley, "Guidelines for Forecasting the Vector-Borne Disease Implications of Water Resources Development." *PEEM Guidelines, No. 2*, Ed. PEEM Secretariat, 2nd ed., WHO/CWS/91.3 (World Health Organization, Geneva 1991). 6J C Bhatia, "The Narmada Valley Project." in-*Health Implications of Public Policy*, Ed. B Ghosh. (Indian Institute of Management, Bangalore 1991).

7 World Health Organization Commission on Health and Environment, "Our Planet, Our Health." (World Health Organization, Geneva 1992).

8 G Surtees, D I H Simpson, E T W Bowen, and W E Grainger, "Ricefield development and arbovirus epidemiology, Kano Plain, Kenya." *Trans R Soc Trop Med Hyg.* 1970, 64:4:511-518.

9 N N Dukhanina, M K Nushin, N I Polevoi, G K Yakubi, and H M Artemev, "The malaria problem and malaria control measures in northern Afganistan. First report. Malaria in northern Afganistan. [In Russian, English summary]." *Med Parazitol Parazit Bolezni.* 1975, 44:338-344.

10 M H Coosemans, "Comparison de l'endemie malarienne dans une zone de riziculture et dans une zone de culture de cotton dans la plaine de la Rusizi, Burundi." *Ann Soc Belge Med Trop.* 1985, 65:supplement 2:187-200.

11 S K Ault, "Effect of demographic patterns, social structure, and human behaviour on malaria." in-*Demography and Vector-Borne Diseases, Ed. M W Service.* (CRC Press, Florida 1989).

12 L E Small, "Irrigation financing policies to promote improved operations and maintenance: the role of the farmer." in-*Selected Working Papers Prepared for the 3rd, 4th, 5th and 6th Meeting of the WHO/FAO/UNEP Panel of experts on Environmental Management for Vector Control (PEEM)., Ed. R Bos.* VBC/87.3 (World Health Organisation, Geneva 1987).

13 J P Doumenge, K E Mott, C Cheung, D Villenave, O Chapuis, M F Perrin, and G Reaud-Thomas, "Atlas of the Global Distibution of Schistosomiasis." (World Health Organization, Geneva 1987).

14 F H Meskal, and H Kloos, "Vector-borne disease occurrence and spread as affected by labor migrations to irrigation schemes in Ethiopia." in-*Demography and Vector-Borne Diseases, Ed. M W Service.* (CRC Press, Florida 1989).

15 E O Adekolu-John, "The impact of lake creation on guinea-worm transmission in Nigeria on the eastern side of Kainji Lake." *Int J Parasit.* 1983, 13:5:427-432.

16 International Rice Research Institute, "Vector-borne Disease Control in Humans Through Rice Agroecosystem Management." (International Rice Research Institute, Manila 1988).

17 C A Pearson, "Awareness of onchocerciasis." *The Lancet.* 1986, 331:8510:805-806.

18 H I Shuval, "Wastewater Irrigation in Developing Countries: Health Effects and Technical Solutions." *Water and Sanitation Discussion Paper Series, No. 2,* (The International Bank for Reconstruction and Development, Washington 1990).

19 H I Shuval, A Adin, B Fattal, E Rawitz, and P Yekutiel, "Wastewater Irrigation in Developing Countries – Health Effects and Technical Solutions." (1986) World Bank, Washington. Integrated Resource Recovery No 6: World Bank Technical Paper No 51.

20 R H Meakins, Personal communication.

21 Environmental Resources Ltd, "Environmental Health Impact Assessment of Irrigated Agricultural Development Projects." (December 1983) World Health Organization Europe.

chapter 8

FISHERIES HEALTH HAZARDS AND THE PROJECT STAGE AT WHICH SAFEGUARDS MAY BE REQUIRED

Project stage	Health hazard	Examples and causes
Location	Communicable Disease	Contact with disease foci, pollution of water sources
	Non-Communicable Disease	Pollution, algal blooms
	Injury	Storm and flood, drowning
Planning and Design	Communicable Disease	Use of excreta and sewage as fertilizer
	Malnutrition	Loss of common property resources
Construction	Communicable Disease	Poor sanitation, water supply and food hygiene, STDs, exposure to vectors
	Non-Communicable Disease	Inadequate occupational safety measures, drowning
	Injury	Inadequate occupational safety measures
Operation	Communicable Disease	Food poisoning, poor monitoring of water for pathogens and toxins, poor processing standards, creation of vector breeding sites
	Non-Communicable Disease	Misuse of chemicals, antibiotics, fish poisons, Respiratory diseases associated with fish processing
	Malnutrition	Loss of common property resources
	Injury	Storm and flood, drowning, cuts, lacerations and infections following injuries

This section includes fresh and salt water, capture and culture fisheries (aquaculture). The reliance on fresh water and marine animal life as a source of food is increasing. All fisheries can involve substantial post-harvest processing in the form of gutting, peeling, slicing, canning, freezing and cooking. Processing occurs both on land and at sea. The occupational health and safety of such industrial processes requires separate attention.

1   MARINE CAPTURE FISHERIES

1.1   COMMUNICABLE DISEASE

Marine organisms can contain parasites which cause serious human disease. Quality control is essential to ensure the safety of aquatic produce during preparation and processing. Rejection of shipments from developing countries can have catastrophic effects on producers. Contamination can occur at many stages. After capture, produce must be cleaned, gutted, refrigerated and stored.

The habit of eating raw or partially cooked aquatic organisms is increasing among some communities.

EXAMPLES

◆ Peeling of shrimps is the process which affords the greatest risk of *Salmonella* contamination[1].

◆ The change in eating habits of some Indonesians to eating raw or half-cooked sea food has resulted in an increase in anisakiasis[2].

◆ An epidemic of cholera swept through South America in 1991 with over 533,000 cases[3]. The bacterium was probably introduced to Peru by shipping[4]. The primary infections were probably from eating raw sea food. Subsequent spread was due to unchlorinated and contaminated water supplies[4]. Chlorination had ceased because of a miscalculated risk of cancer[4]. Additional factors included illegal water connection, drinking unboiled water, contaminated domestic storage of water and illegal diversion of sewage to vegetable plots[3].

1.2   NON-COMMUNICABLE DISEASE

Marine fish and shellfish are susceptible to contamination by natural toxins produced by certain algae. The problem is most acute when algal blooms occur. These are referred to as "red tides" and may be caused by excess agricultural runoff. The problem is worldwide and associated with both fresh and sea waters[5]. The algae kill fish and render molluscs and crustaceans toxic. The toxins can cause paralytic shellfish poisoning. Children are especially vulnerable because their toxic thresholds are very low.

In aquaculture developments, monitoring of harmful algal species is crucial for public health purposes but must not replace testing of produce for biotoxins. Site location can be crucial.

Ciguatera is a severe neurotoxin sometimes harboured by certain Pacific and Caribbean reef fish. It originates in plankton and is concentrated in the food chain. Fear of poisoning severely restricts fish exports from several island nations. Outbreaks also disrupt the tourist industry. Ciguatoxic biotopes can be created by development activities that disrupt the reef system. These include the construction of hotels, aircraft runways and wharves[6].

Processing of sea-food, particularly crabs, has been associated with increased prevalence of chronic obstructive airways disease among the workforce[7].

1.3 MALNUTRITION

Fishing communities are often impoverished and dependent on a variable resource. Aquaculture development can cause economic shifts or changes in access to resources that may disturb basic household nutrition.

1.4 INJURY

Fishing and aquaculture can be hazardous occupations with exposure to extreme environments and danger of drowning.

The World Bank publication: Occupational Health and Safety Guidelines[8], notes that there are many complex safety issues associated with fishing and the design of fishing vessels. These include asphyxia due to the release of gases by rotting fish. Falls and machinery are the most common causes of injury at sea[9]. The fishing industry is notorious for the risk of injury death, through drowning and other hazards. This is particularly so in coastal countries.

2 MARINE CULTURE FISHERIES

2.1 COMMUNICABLE DISEASE

The pollution by human excreta of waters used for harvesting shellfish can be the source of many enteric infections. Molluscs, particularly bivalves, are frequently grown in waters contaminated by excreta and can accumulate pathogens.

Some species of mosquitoes are especially adapted to brackish water habitats. Consequently, coastal ponds can become important breeding sites for vectors such as malaria mosquitoes.

EXAMPLES

◆ An epidemic of shell-fish borne hepatitis A in China in 1988 affected 292,000 persons and was related to the consumption of contaminated clams[10].

◆ Brackish coastal fish ponds and lagoons in Indonesia are important breeding sites of malaria mosquitoes when they are covered with an algal mat or abandoned.

2.2 NON-COMMUNICABLE DISEASE

Many waters in which shellfish are harvested are polluted by domestic and industrial wastes from which bivalves can accumulate potentially toxic chemical contaminants.

The potential human health hazard associated with the use of antibiotics in intensive fish production is a matter of current debate. *See also Livestock, chapter 10.* Many countries now refuse to import shellfish which have been treated with antibiotics.

EXAMPLE

◆ Export of Philippine shrimp to Japan is severely affected by Japanese inspection for antibiotic contamination, according to The Philippine Star, April 28, 1992.

2.3 MALNUTRITION

In Ecuador large areas of mangrove forest along the coast have been destroyed as entrepreneurs have constructed saltwater fish ponds for shrimp farming. The displaced people have been marginalised and have lost their independent food security. For a while some worked on the fish farms but now the source of fry from the sea has been exhausted and the fish farms are failing. Meanwhile the area is no longer capable of producing food for the indigenous population[11].

3 FRESHWATER CAPTURE FISHERIES

3.1 NON-COMMUNICABLE DISEASE

Biotoxins produced by algal blooms can seriously affect fish production. *See Marine Capture Fisheries section 1.2.*

3.2 MALNUTRITION

In river deltas, such as the Ganges and Brahamaputra in Bangladesh, annual flooding provides an opportunity for intensive fishing. The landless poor, in particular, derive a substantial part of their nutritional needs from their rights to fish the flooded lands. Development projects that are designed to restrict flooding can alter migratory routes and spawning grounds and deprive the poor of these fish.

4   FRESHWATER CULTURE FISHERIES

Freshwater fish production could play an important role in increasing food production. However the changes to the environment and interaction with other development projects can have harmful effects on the health of local people.

Freshwater fisheries are developed in ponds, reservoirs, rice paddies and irrigation canals.

TABLE I   Positive and negative effects of fish culture on health in the Sahel (adapted from USAID[12]).

Positive	Negative

Improved nutrition leading to:
    increased survival,
    better physical and mental growth,
    increased resistance to disease,
    increased productivity and vigour
	New breeding sites for vectors of malaria, schistosomiasis and dracunculiasis

	Contamination of water with human and animal waste
Improved cash income	Transmission of amoebic and bacillary dysentery, intestinal worms, cholera
Attraction of settlers	Contamination with pesticide runoff
Contribution to successful integrated rural development	Conflict with livestock and forestry projects

4.1   COMMUNICABLE DISEASE

Two main areas of concern are pathogens from wastewater reuse and creation of, or increase in, vector breeding sites.

Human and animal excreta can provide a valuable source of fertilizer for fish ponds. The technique has been practised successfully in Germany for many years. Sewage waste stabilization ponds are also used. However fish, fish products and fishponds can easily become contaminated with pathogens which may affect workers, processors and consumers. Treatment and monitoring is required to minimise health risks.

EXAMPLES

◆ Infection with *Clonorchis sinensis*, the Chinese liver fluke, is increasing in Taiwan. The increase in the popularity of eating raw fish, the new policy of raising pigs close to local fish ponds and farmers eating the fish uncooked are considered responsible[2].

◆ In NE Thailand, raw fish eating is widespread and there is a correspondingly high prevalence rate for the associated parasitic diseases.

Pathogen removal must occur in pretreatment processes and during use. Thereafter, aquaculture produce must be treated for pathogen removal. Pretreatment of raw sewage by 8–10 day detention in anaerobic ponds is required to remove settleable pathogens. Nightsoil should be stored for two weeks before use. A stable plankton community should be established before fish stocking. Loading of wastewater into fish ponds must be suspended for two weeks prior to harvest. Harvested fish must be held in clean water to evacuate their guts. Threshold concentrations of bacteria in fish muscle must not be exceeded. *Salmonella* concentration should be zero[1]. In some regions there is a risk of parasite transmission such as *Paragonimus*, *Diphyllobothrium* and *Opisthorchis*.

Small dams are built for many reasons including fish farming, small hydropower generation, irrigation and water supply. They are often built informally, to low standards and to meet local needs, and are not recorded in any inventory[13]. In Africa they provide breeding sites for vectors such as malaria mosquitoes and schistosomiasis snails. In India and Pakistan fish ponds could breed malaria mosquitoes although the water may often be too contaminated.

EXAMPLE

◆ In Nigeria, the surface area of small impoundments is at least 3.5 times, and the shoreline at least 10 times that of large dams. In Zimbabwe there are between 10,000 and 20,000 farm dams. In Nyanza province, Kenya, some 50,000 small impoundments were created in 3 years during the late 50's[13].

This Kenyan rice farmer is eating
maize and beans. Changes from
subsistence to cash crops may,
paradoxically, increase malnutrition.
This can occur because of shortages of
subsistence foods or because of
unequal entitlements to cash
purchases within the household.

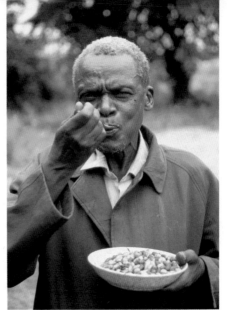

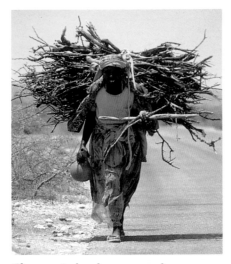

Changes in land use can reduce access
to fuelwood and fodder. A woman in
Somalia has to carry heavy loads for
long distances. This may affect her
posture and nutritional status and
reduce the time available for child
care.

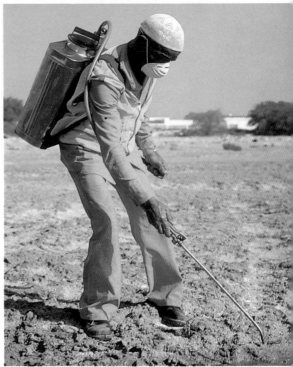

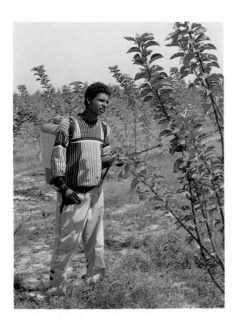

This municipal worker in Dubai is
wearing appropriate protective
clothing for spraying insecticides. His
overalls are washed daily.

Pesticides are often applied by poorly
trained and supervised workers
without protective clothing. This
Egyptian operator risks both acute and
chronic poisoning.

In the Republic of Benin, open wells are cheaper to install and easier to maintain than handpumps. In this example a lid was provided to stop children and animals from falling in. However, the water is easily contaminated by dirty containers and ropes.

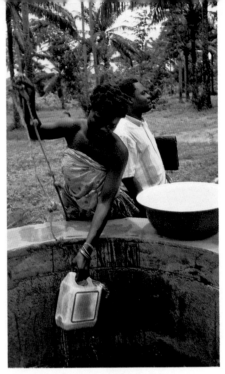

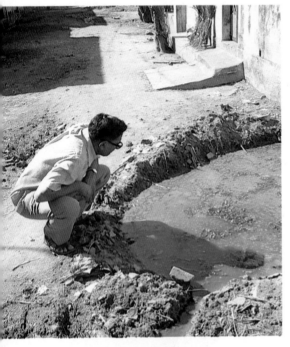

Piped water supplies are often installed in urban houses without adequate provision for waste water disposal. In this town in Southern India, foul water accumulates in shallow open pits and breeds mosquitoes that transmit filariasis. Other breeding sites include open drains blocked by domestic solid waste.

The ventilated pit latrine was invented here, at the Blair Research Laboratory in Zimbabwe. It uses natural drafts, light and shade to remove smells and prevent the breeding of filth flies and mosquitoes. It can play a significant role in reducing open defecation.

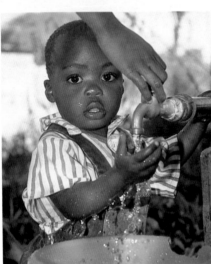

Clean water delivery can assist in the prevention of childhood diarrhoeas. However, proper maintenance is often difficult.

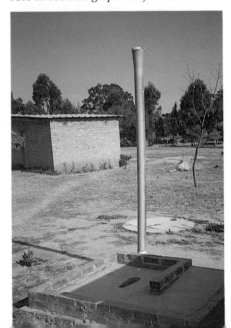

This community in Thailand has been displaced by a dam project. They were resettled and provided with a rubber plantation at the forest edge in place of their subsistence agriculture. As malaria mosquitoes in that region breed in shaded streams at the forest edge, the choice of resettlement site was questionable.

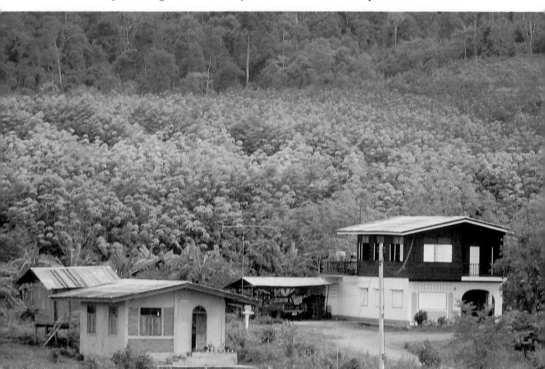

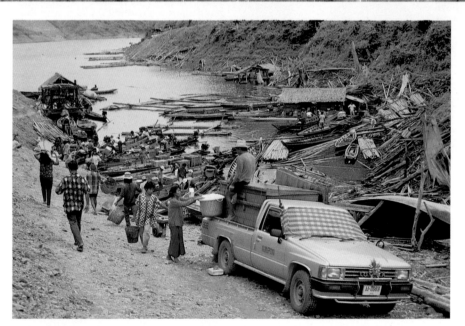

Many different communities are affected by a development project. This new reservoir in Thailand attracted fishing folk from distant river basins. They were living in an insanitary informal settlement at the reservoir margin.

This child is labouring in a turquoise factory in Jaipur, India. Child labour is all too common. Such children are educationally deprived, poorly paid and exposed to many health hazards.

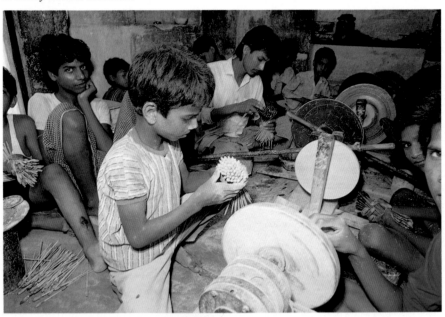

Many women are engaged in heavy construction work, such as this bricklayer in Botswana. They are exposed to gender specific health hazards, such as miscarriage, and may also be subjected to sexual harassment.

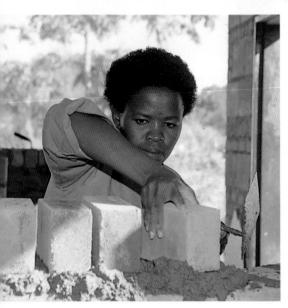

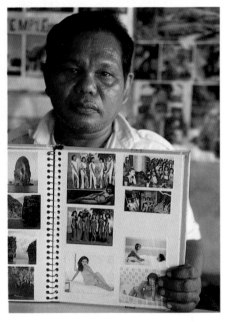

Professional sex workers are at considerable risk of sexually transmitted diseases. A hotel bell captain, in Thailand, displays a selection of "masseurs" as an alternative to site seeing tours.

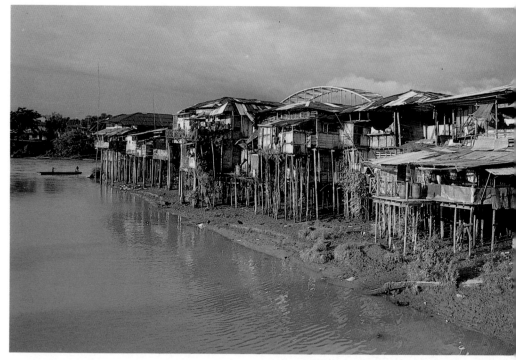

Rapid urbanization has led to the proliferation of shanty towns such as this one on the San Juan river, Istmina, Colombia. Such dwellings are built in hazardous locations subject to flood, fire or landslide. They are often inadequately supplied with drinking water and sanitation.

Solid waste disposal is a major problem in many cities. Many people gain their livelihoods from recycling waste. They are vital to the life of the city but are often very poor and very young. These children are working on "Smokey Mountain" in Manila. They are exposed to hazardous materials and risk injuries, infections and skin disorders.

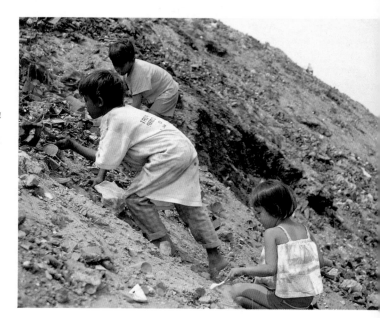

Forestry work has a high injury rate. Unskilled workers frequently operate hazardous machinery without adequate protection. This bare-footed chain-saw operator was cutting logs for a multinational operator on the Gogol River, Papua New Guinea.

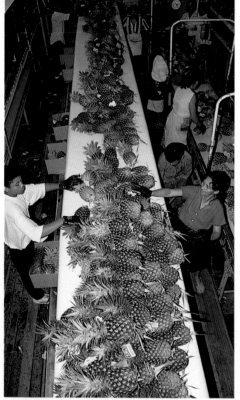

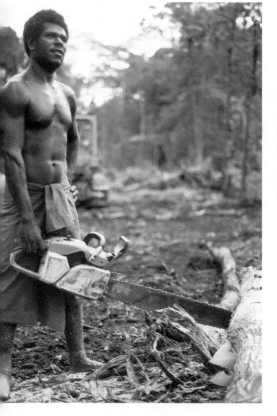

Agricultural processing industries expose workers to health hazards such as acidic liquids and irritant dusts. These workers, in Honduras, are well protected by rubber gloves.

This damaged bus was photographed in Papua New Guinea. The high risk of traffic injuries is an important feature of transport projects in less developed countries.

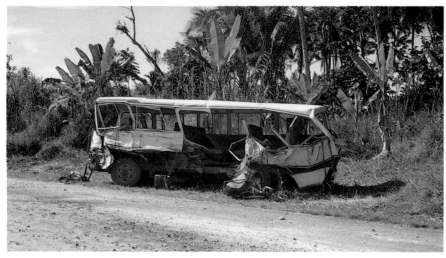

Dust induced lung disease is a common occupational health hazard. This woman is wearing a home-made face mask as meagre protection against cotton fibre in a Bangladeshi garment factory. Preventive measures are frequently inadequate.

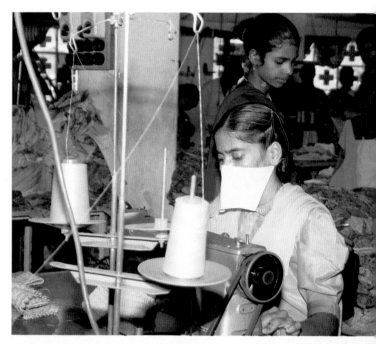

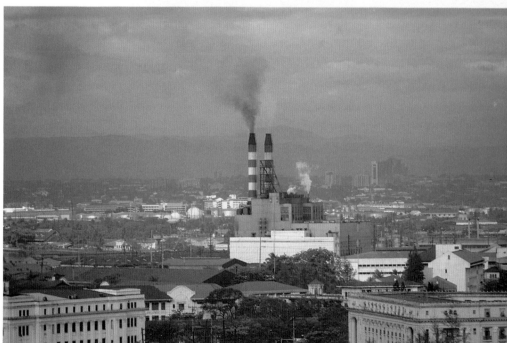

This fossil-fuel fired power station is emitting particulates and other pollutants into the already smog laden atmosphere of Manila, Philippines. Polluted air significantly increases the risk of respiratory disease.

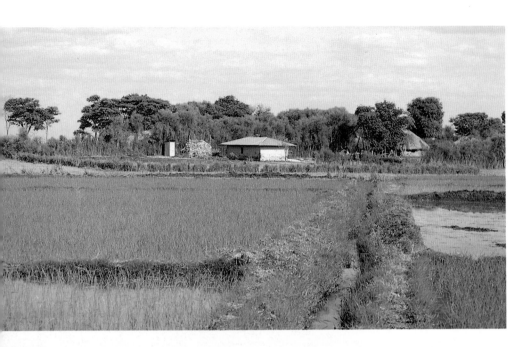

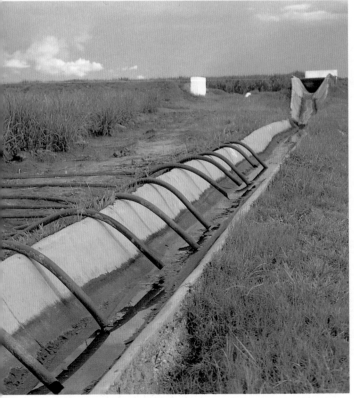

Poorly maintained irrigation
ditches create stagnant
waters harbouring malaria
mosquitoes and bilharzia
snails. Families living close
to the scheme, such as this
household in Kenya, are
most vulnerable.

A well-maintained
sugarcane irrigation system
in Zambia. The absence of
standing water deters
malaria mosquitoes and
bilharzia snails.

The health hazard represented by large numbers of small reservoirs is likely to be very great because of the total area and shoreline that they represent.

Fish ponds become mosquito breeding sites when they are poorly managed. Good management involves removal of surface and emergent aquatic vegetation which provides shelter for mosquito larvae.

A new health hazard to tilapia hatchery workers in the Philippines has emerged with a change in breeding technique. Workers now spend longer wading in the ponds and suffer from an increase in foot infections[1].

4.2 NON-COMMUNICABLE DISEASE/INJURY

Water can easily be contaminated with trace metals, pesticides, disinfectants, antibiotics and hormones.

When wastewater is reused for agriculture, industrial effluent must be carefully monitored for toxic chemicals and metals. Culture of molluscs in wastewater systems is not advisable because of bio-accumulation of contaminants[1].

Fish poisons such as phosgene producing chemicals are frequently used to harvest fish and are potentially lethal to people if wrongly handled.

5 REFERENCES

1 R S V Pullin, H Rosenthal, and Maclean J L Ed., "Aquaculture and Environment in Developing Countries." *ICLAM Conference Proceedings 31.* (ICLAM, Manila 1991).

2 J H Cross, and K D Murrell, "The 33rd SEAMEO-TROPMED regional seminar on emerging problems in food-borne parasitic zoonoses: impact on agriculture and public health." *Southeast Asian J Trop Med Public Health.* 1991, 22:1:4–15.

3 D L Swerdlow, E D Mintz, M Rodriguez, E Tejada, C Ocampo, L Espejo, K D Greene, W Saldana, L Seminario, R V Tauxe, J W Wells, N H Bean, A A Ries, M Pollack, B Vertiz, and P A Blake, "Waterborne transmission of epidemic cholera in Trujillo, Peru: lessons for a continent at risk." *The Lancet.* 1992, 340:8810:28–32.

4 C Anderson, "Cholera epidemic traced to risk miscalculation." *Nature.* 1991, 354:28 Nov:255.

5 J M Dunlop, "Blooming algae." *Brit Med J.* 1991, 302:671–672.

6 N D Lewis, "Disease and development: ciguatera fish poisoning." *Soc Sci Med.* 1986, 23:10:983–993.

7 R R Orford, and J T Wilson, "Epidemiologic and immunologic studies in processors of the king crab." *Am J Ind Med.* 1985, 7:155–169.

8 The World Bank, "Occupational Health and Safety Guidelines." (The World Bank Environment Department, Washington 1988).

9 World Health Organization Commission on Health and Environment, "Our Planet, Our Health." (World Health Organization, Geneva 1992).

10 World Health Organization, "Report of the Food and Agriculture Panel." (1991) World Health Organization Commission on Health and the Environment. Unpublished.
11 Television Trust for the Environment, "Shrimp Fever." (Channel 4 Television, London 1992).
12 Family Health Care Inc./USAID, "Health Impact Guidelines for the Design of Development Projects in the Sahel: Volume 1: Sector-Specific Reviews and Methodology." (13 April 1979) United States Agency for International Development, Washington. PN-AAJ-381.
13 J M Jewsbury, and A M A Imevbore, "Small dam health studies." *Parasit Today.* 1988, 4:2:57–59.

chapter 9

FORESTRY HEALTH HAZARDS AND THE PROJECT STAGE AT WHICH SAFEGUARDS MAY BE REQUIRED

Project stage	Health hazard	Examples and causes
Location	Communicable Disease	Contact with disease foci
	Non-Communicable Disease	Loss of potential medicinal plants
	Malnutrition	Loss of common property resources
Planning and design	Communicable Disease	Resettlement, disruption of water supplies
	Malnutrition	Loss of common property resources
Operation	Communicable Disease	Logging camps, poor sanitation, water supply and food hygiene, STDs, exposure to vectors, colonization of vectors
	Malnutrition	Loss of food, fodder and fuelwood
	Injury	Hearing loss, poor occupational safety, bites, stings, infections following injuries; transport crashes and collisions, fractures

This chapter is concerned with deforestation, reafforestation, tree crop plantations and development of forest reserves. It intends to address these issues at project level rather than contributing to the debate on global environmental change. It is concerned with the health hazards experienced by communities in areas where trees are, were, or will become a dominant plant form.

See also Cross-Cutting Issues, chapter 2, Changes in Land Use and Resettlement; and Agriculture, chapter 6, Plantation Agriculture.

1   COMMUNICABLE DISEASE

The effect of deforestation and reafforestation on vector-borne disease is complex and should always be considered when planning development projects. Much of the following account is from a recent review[1].

1.1   ARBOVIRUSES

Over 520 arboviruses are known of which about 100 cause human disease[2]. The vectors include mosquitoes and ticks. There is often a natural cycle of transmission between forest dwelling animals and vectors. People become infected when they penetrate the forest and they may then carry the infection to human settlements. There is a risk that previously uninfected vectors may then commence transmission of the arbovirus in villages and towns. Alternatively, settlement of forest clearings and disturbance of natural environments may expose workers and their dependents to infection.

EXAMPLES

◆ In West Africa, yellow fever spread to human communities primarily from forest penetration but forest clearance by the logging industry was probably also important[3,4].

◆ Kyasanur Forest Disease, in Southern India, is a serious febrile illness transmitted by ticks. An epidemic occurred quite suddenly during the late 1950's with a 5% fatality rate. The epidemic was explained by human disturbance of the forest and the conjunction of monkeys, cattle, ticks and an invasive plant[5,6,7].

1.2   MALARIA

In tropical Africa, the main malaria vectors live in both forest and savannah. The most important vector has many genetic forms which are believed to be of different efficacy in malaria transmission. These genetic forms are associated with different environments and especially the change from forest to savannah[1].

In South America and South East Asia the most important malaria is associated with forests[1]. Indigenous forest dwellers tend to have high levels of immunity. There is a natural stability that is disrupted by forest disturbance. Epidemics occur when non-immune people migrate to the forest and forest fringe.

EXAMPLE

◆ In Brazil some 80–90% of malaria is registered from the Amazon basin[8]. This has largely been the result of recent colonization[9]. Large increases in malaria cases have been registered in forest towns[10]. Each year, along the Transamazon highways, some 5–25% of the population contract malaria. During the 1970s malaria represented some 40–50% of admissions to hospitals associated with the highways. The malaria affecting migrant settlers is a different species to that found in indigenous peoples. Malaria is considered an important factor in the reduction of crop yields.

In forest areas of South East Asia malaria is transmitted by mosquitoes breeding in two separate habitats. Where mosquitoes breed in deeply shaded pools or streams, malaria transmission is associated with sojourn in the forest and affects small groups of people, such as forestry workers. Other mosquitoes breed in partially shaded or sunlit water. Such breeding sites occur at the forest fringe or as a result of forest disturbance and deforestation. Deforestation removes the shade loving mosquitoes. Plantation crops favour the partial shade or sunlit loving species. Large groups of people may be affected and epidemics occur. Resettlement schemes should consider siting new settlements as far as possible from the forest.

EXAMPLES

◆ Between 1960 and 1980 much forest in SE Thailand was destroyed by logging and cassava plantations and malaria declined. Since 1980, there has been a rapid increase in tree crops such as coffee and rubber and malaria morbidity has increased. The virtual disappearance of severe malaria could be reversed by the government's successful promotion of tree crops[1].

◆ Cyclical malaria epidemics in Malaysia over a period of some fifty years were correlated with rubber replanting in response to market fluctuations[11,12]. The vector breeds in sunlit streams exposed by tree clearing.

In Peninsular Malaysia and Java, destruction of coastal swamp forest and mangroves adversely affected the prevalence of malaria. The brackish water zone was relatively free of malaria as long as the mangroves remained undisturbed. However, they were cut for charcoal, mine props or to establish fish ponds. The sunlit, brackish water favoured an important malaria mosquito[1]. The Indonesian transmigration programme has moved large numbers of non-immune people from Java to the outer islands. New settlements are sited in previously forested areas. Land preparation includes clear-felling and burning of forest and this eliminates the forest vector. However, migrants are still at risk from malaria when they overnight in the forest in search of fuelwood, food and medicinal plants. In some areas, a different vector has successfully colonised the cleared lands[1]. In Sri Lanka, epidemic malaria corresponded with the period of forest clearance. Deforestation and tea planting led to massive soil erosion. Perennial rivers were scoured and flow became erratic. The malaria mosquito bred in stream pools in otherwise dry rivers. This led to the apparent anomaly of severe epidemic malaria among non-immune populations during drought years[1].

In Indochina generally, a severe drug resistant malaria has evolved in the disturbed forests and this is now spreading throughout the region[13].

In Trinidad, during the 1940s, malaria became a serious problem when forest clearance made way for cocoa plantations. The ecological linkage was complex. Shade trees were planted to protect young cocoa plantations from excessive sunlight. The shade trees created mosquito breeding sites in the leaf axils of epiphytic bromeliads and malaria outbreaks occurred. The epidemic was controlled when the nurse trees were reduced and plantation techniques modified[14].

1.3   LEISHMANIASIS

In the Amazon basin, there are several different species of the *Leishmania* parasite and several different sandfly vectors. Many of the parasites have wild animals as primary hosts. Environmental change can readily contribute to epidemics. Cutaneous leishmaniasis is commonly associated with forest occupations but large-scale developments have frequently produced outbreaks among communities of labourers. Settlements near the forest edge have also been affected.

EXAMPLES

♦ Many labourers suffered from cutaneous leishmaniasis during construction of Sao Paulo state railway in Brazil in 1908[1].

♦ In 1970 large areas of native forest were cleared in Monte Dourado, Brazil, for planting with gmelina and pine forests. Twelve years later it was shown that a sandfly vector of cutaneous leishmaniasis and a rat that is an important reservoir host had adapted well to the forest plantation. The form of leishmaniasis involved can be incurable and highly mutilating. There is concern that increased outbreaks of the disease will occur[15].

Visceral leishmaniasis, by contrast, is more frequently associated with drier areas and is extending its range into the Amazon Basin with the destruction of the forest. Both the vector sandfly and the fox reservoir have adapted well to the peridomestic environment.

1.4   CHAGAS' DISEASE

This incurable disease is transmitted by triatomine bugs in South and Central America. There are many animal hosts. The original habitat was woodland but the vector adapted to human habitations and deforested areas. With the widespread destruction of forest since Columbian times, the disease has become widespread. The disease has not been a major problem in the Amazon forest but there is a real danger that either sylvatic vectors will become adapted to the domiciliary habit or that common domestic vectors will spread into cleared areas. The parasite is commonly found in forest opossums that adapt well to forest disturbance and human compounds.

1.5   FILARIASIS

Other vector-borne diseases associated with forests are loiasis, in West Africa, onchocerciasis, in Africa and America, and Brugian filariasis in Malaysia, Borneo and Sumatra[1]. Loiasis appears to decline where forests are cleared for agriculture but may still be associated with tree crop plantations. Brugian filariasis in South East Asia has an animal reservoir and an association with swamp forest. Particular health risks occur in Malaysian rubber estate workers and their dependents. The rubber estates are surrounded by forest and are commonly invaded by infected monkeys and the mosquito vector[16]. Finally, onchocerciasis in Africa has a complex relationship with savannahs and forests and the disease is usually more severe in savannahs. Deforestation favours the savannah forms while the associated erratic stream flow provides breeding sites for the vector blackfly.

1.6   SCHISTOSOMIASIS

Schistosomiasis is a widespread disease with an aquatic snail host. In Africa, a pathogenic species appears to be spreading into new areas as they become deforested and invaded by the snail. In the Philippines, the snail host favours shaded habitats of the flood plain forest and is usually absent from well-tended rice paddy[17]. In Sulawesi, there is concern that the disease could spread as forest cover is reduced.

1.7   SLEEPING SICKNESS

The risk of human African trypanosomiasis is generally reducing in parallel with the destruction of savannah and riverine woodland. However in some areas the tsetse fly vector has colonised plantations of cocoa, coffee and oil palms. Recrudescence of the disease may occur if infected migrant labour introduces the parasite[18].

2   NON-COMMUNICABLE DISEASE

A major factor in the concern about deforestation relates to the species richness and genetic diversity of tropical forests.

Forests contain unknown numbers of potentially valuable medicinal plants and animals. In industrialised countries some 50% of all drug preparations are derived from natural products. Many of these drugs are extremely complex and unlikely to be synthesised by chance in the laboratory[19]. The value of medicinal drugs derived from wild species of plants is believed to exceed US$50 billion per year[20]. Although medicinal plants may provide specific cures to communicable as well as non-communicable diseases, the anti-cancer properties are of particular interest.

EXAMPLES

◆ Of some 3,000 plants that were shown to have activity against cancer cells, some 70% were derived from tropical forests[20].

◆ One of the world's major pharmaceutical companies, Merck, entered an agreement to pay a Costa Rican conservation organisation US$1 million plus royalties for the right to search for new medicines in local forests[21].

---

3   MALNUTRITION

See also Agriculture, chapter 6, Plantation Agriculture.

Forestry projects change community access to forest produce: food, fuel, fodder and other products. Commercial forestry decreases access, or leads to deforestation, or establishes monocultures. Replacement of grazing areas and multispecies forests with monoculture plantations may cause a decrease in available fodder or forest foods for human consumption.

EXAMPLES

◆ In one area in Himachal Pradesh, India, a natural forest of mixed hardwoods was replaced with managed eucalyptus stands for a pulp mill. A combination of decreased access to the forest and reduced grass and green leaf fodder availability, meant that the number of cattle able to be kept per family dropped from seven to one or two[22].

◆ In addition eucalyptus wood burnt unevenly, spitting dangerously due to the oil. It did not provide the same steady, even heat necessary for cooking as did the hardwoods[22].

The logging industry frequently does not implement replacement planting programmes and this has long term implications for food security[23].

For children in particular, foraging in the forest may provide vital supplements of minerals and vitamins to their staple diet. Fodder is collected to feed milch cattle or other animals and the milk provides extra food supplements. Forests can also produce substantial quantities of fodder for domestic animals. However, changing the species of forest trees can reduce their suitability for cattle fodder[24].

EXAMPLE

◆ In Botswana, cattle may derive 50% of their food intake from browsing trees and shrubs[24].

Where labourers or farmers maintain home gardens for food production, the impact of tree crop projects on community food security is reduced. Community forest projects can increase and safeguard forest access.

Trees are an integral part of food security strategies for rural people[25]. Tree ownership provides savings and security; an asset which can offset sudden contingencies such as the cost of ill health[26]. Trees are almost invariably incorporated in production systems where farmers have lived for extended periods. Their value is enhanced in savannah parklands, where most tree cover has been removed. Recent initiatives from FAO have sought to create linkages between foresters and nutritionists[27].

EXAMPLES

◆ In forested areas of northern Thailand 60% of all food, 40 different products, including nuts, roots and berries, comes from the forests.

◆ Communities living near forest in Nigeria obtained 84% of their animal protein from bushmeat.

◆ In Peru the national average of those eating bushmeat, including those who live far from forest land, is 41%[25].

Fuelwood is essential for releasing the nutrients in food through cooking, processing and preserving surplus food supplies. Where fuelwood is scarce, food and time are also likely to be scarce. Fuelwood collection makes substantial demands on women's time. Less time may then be spent cooking and food may be more easily contaminated, increasing disease incidence. Less time may be available for child care. Where fuel is scarce families may eat one instead of two cooked meals per day, or use non-boiled water, or use foods that cook quickly but contain less nutrients[28]. *See also Energy, chapter 5.*

Transportation of heavy fuelwood loads for long distances is likely to have a detrimental effect on women's nutritional energy balance. It may be a major factor in malnutrition and a major contributor to the shortage of labour for farming. The task of gathering fuelwood and water may consume 400–500 calories/day out of an already inadequate intake[30].

EXAMPLES

◆ Women in rural areas of south India purchase fuelwood to save time for other tasks even though this reduces their disposable income[29].

◆ A study in India suggested that the energy cost of collecting fuelwood, water and other domestic chores represented nearly one third of a woman's daily expenditure[29].

◆ In several African cities poor families have to spend 20–30% of their income on charcoal[30].

Deforestation has a major effect on agriculture by disrupting the supply of water to irrigation systems. Large scale deforestation in major rivers can cause flooding in fertile downstream areas destroying life and means of food security[31].

The species richness and genetic diversity of tropical forests indicate that they may contain important new food plants. At present 85% of the world's food supply derives from only 8 plant species and within these species genetic diversity has consistently been reduced. The genetic diversity of wild plants may be vital for conferring resistance to insect attack and plant disease. In the Amazonian region of Brazil, wild or spontaneous populations of at least 50 perennial crops are at risk from deforestation[33].

EXAMPLES

◆ In Leyte, Philippines, a flood reported to have been caused by deforestation killed 7,000 and made 120,000 people homeless during 1991 (The Nation, Bangkok, 12 November 1991).

◆ In Maharastra, India, deforestation is reputed to be responsible for drying up the water supplies of 23,000 villages[32].

◆ In Papua New Guinea there are 251 known species of tree with edible fruit but only 17% are cultivated. The winged bean, *Psophocarpus tetragonolobus*, is grown in over 50 countries but before the 1970's it was confined to forest peoples in Papua New Guinea[34].

---

4 INJURY

The occupational safety record of logging and woodworking industries is often poor[35]. Hill logging operations involve many dangerous procedures. Most of the labour force are local contract workers with little education or experience of the hazards. The labour force may live in poor accommodation in logging camps with inadequate food and sanitation. They may be overworked so that accumulated fatigue contributes to low efficiency and high injury rates. Logging trucks are often overloaded and logging roads poorly constructed. Woodworking machinery is fast moving and dangerous, especially where guards are inadequate.

Noise from equipment such as chain-saws can effect hearing and cause hearing loss as well as stress and behavioural problems[31].

Forestry workers are also susceptible to injuries from animal bites (including snakes) with the risk of infections, including rabies and tetanus. They are also exposed to plant poisonings and stings.

Deforestation and commercial forestry increase the distance that local communities must travel to obtain fuelwood. Long journeys bearing heavy loads lead to back and other muscoskeletal injuries. Women may be especially vulnerable.

EXAMPLE

♦ In Sarawak 73% of industrial injuries were recorded from the logging and woodworking industries during 1979. Of some 20,000 workers, 5% were injured and 0.25% were killed. The industry death rate was twenty times higher than Canada's[35].

♦ Between 1966 and 1981 the distance travelled in northern Uganda to find fuelwood increased from an average of 0.9km to 4.4km[36].

---

5   REFERENCES

1   J F Walsh, D H Molyneux, and M H Birley, "Deforestation: effects on vector-borne disease." *Parasitology.* 1993, 106:55–75.

2   S Morse, and A Schluederberg, "Emerging viruses: the evolution of viruses and viral diseases." *J Infect Dis.* 1990, 162:1–7.

3   A J Haddow, K C Smithburn, and A F Mahaffy, "Monkeys in relation to yellow fever in Bwamba Country, Uganda." *Trans R Soc Trop Med hyg.* 1947, 40:677–700.

4   R N T W Fiennes, "Zoonoses and the Origins and Ecology of Human Disease." (Academic Press, London 1978).

5   H Hoogstraal, "Ticks in relation to human diseases caused by viruses." *Ann Rev Entomol.* 1966, 11:261–308.

6   H Hoogstraal, "Changing patterns of tick-borne diseases in modern society." *Ann Rev Entomol.* 1981, 26:75–99.

7   M J Boshell, "Kyasanur forest disease: ecological considerstions." *Am J Trop Med Hyg.* 1969, 18:67–80.

8   C E A Coimbra, "Human factors in the epidemiology of malaria in the Brazilian Amazon." *Hum Org.* 1988, 47:3:254–260.

9   R M Prothero, "Resettlement and health: Amazonia in tropical perspective." in-*A Desordem Ecologia na Amazonica*, (Universidade Federal do Para (UFPA), Belem, Para, Brazil 1991).

10   P B McGreevy, R Dietze, A Prata, and S C Hembree, "Effects of immigration on the prevalence of malaria in rural areas of the Amazon Basin of Peru." *Mem Inst Oswaldo Cruz.* 1989, 84:485–491.

11   M W Service, "The importance of ecological studies on malaria vectors." *Bull Soc Vector Ecol.* 1989, 14:1:26–38.

12   J Singh, and A S Tham, "Case History Of Malaria Vector Control Through The Application Of Environmental Management in Malaysia." (1988) World Health Organisation. WHO/VBC/88.960.

13   V P Sharma, and A V Kondrashin Ed., "Forest Malaria in Southeast Asia, Proceedings of an Informal Consultative Meeting, WHO/MRC, 18–22 February 1991." (World Health Organisation, New Delhi 1991).

14   W G Downs, and C S Pittendrigh, "Bromeliad malaria in Trinidad, British West Indies." *Am J Trop Med Hyg.* 1949, 26:47–66.

15   R Lainson, "Demographic changes and their influence on the epidemiology of the American Leishmaniases." in-*Demography and Vector-Borne Diseases, Ed. M W Service.* (CRC Press, Florida 1989).

16 J W Mak, W H Cheong, P K F Yen, P K C Lin, and W C Chan, "Studies on the epidemiology of sub-periodic *Brugia malayi* in Malaysia: *problems in its control.*" *Acta Tropica.* 1982, 39:237–245.

17 T P Persigan, N G Hairston, J J Jauregui, E G Garcia, R T Santos, B C Santos, and A A Besa, "Studies on *Schistosoma japonicum* infection in the Philippines. 2. The molluscan host." *WHO Bull.* 1958, 18:481–578.

18 A M Jordan, "Man and changing patterns of the African trypanosomiases." in-*Demography and Vector-Borne Diseases, Ed. M W Service.* (CRC Press, Florida 1989).

19 J G Bruhn, "The use of natural products in modern medicine." *Acta Pharm Nord.* 1989, 1:3:117–130.

20 C Bird, "Medicines from the rainforest." *New Scientist.* 1991,

21 L Roberts, "Chemical prospecting: hope for vanishing ecosystems?" *Science.* 1992, 256:5060:1142–3.

22 J Price, Personal communication.

23 R D Mann, "Africa on the brink: Time running out: The urgent need for tree planting in Africa." *The Ecologist.* 1990, 20:2:48–53.

24 R H Meakins, Personal communication.

25 M Hoskins, "The contribution of forestry to food security." *Unasylva.* 1990, 41:3–13.

26 R Chambers, and M Leach, "Trees as savings and security for the rural poor." *Unasylva.* 1990, 41:39–52.

27 C Ogden, "Building nutritional considerations into forestry development efforts." *Unasylva.* 1990, 41:20–28.

28 A Fleuret, "The impact of fuelwood scarcity on dietary patterns: hypotheses for research." *Unasylva.* 1990, 41:29.

29 D E C Cooper Weil, A P Alicbusan, J F Wilson, M R Reich, and D J Bradley, "The Impact of Development Policies on Health: A Review of the Literature." (World Health Organization, Geneva 1990).

30 P Harrison, "The Greening of Africa: Breaking through in the battle for land and food." (Paladin, London 1987).

31 World Health Organization Commission on Health and Environment, "Our Planet, Our Health." (World Health Organization, Geneva 1992).

32 World Rainforest Movement, "Rainforest Destruction: Causes, Effects and False Solutions." (World Rainforest Movement, Penang, Malaysia 1990).

33 N J H Smith, and R E Schultes, "Deforestation and shrinking crop gene-pools in Amazonia." *Environ Conserv.* 1990, 17:227–234.

34 C Caufield, "Tropical Moist Forests: The Resources, The People, The Threat." (Earthscan, London 1982).

35 E Hong, "Natives of Sarawak: Survival in Borneo's Vanishing Forests." (Institut Masyarakat, Pulau Pinang, Malaysia 1987).

36 A C Hamilton, "Deforestation in Uganda." (OUP, Nairobi 1984).

chapter 10

LIVESTOCK

LIVESTOCK RELATED HEALTH HAZARDS AND THE PROJECT STAGE AT WHICH SAFEGUARDS MAY BE REQUIRED

Project stage	Health hazard	Examples and causes
Location	Communicable Disease	Contact with disease foci, water supply
	Malnutrition	Loss of common property resources
Planning and Design	Communicable Disease	Zoonoses, creation of vector habitats, importation of stock, misuse of drugs
	Malnutrition	Environmental degradation
Operation	Communicable Disease	Waste disposal, contamination of water supplies, zoonoses, poor processing and storage, misuse of antibiotics
	Non-Communicable Disease	Chemical residues from contaminated feeds, heavy metals in slurry, misuse of drugs, lung disease
	Malnutrition	Loss of grazing
	Injury	Animal bites, kicks, goring, fractures, cuts and grazes.

1 GENERAL

See also Manufacture and Trade, chapter 12, Leather Tanning and Finishing.

1.1 COMMUNICABLE DISEASE: ZOONOSES

Several communicable diseases can be increased by the importation of exotic breeds of livestock or the intensification of livestock production. Pigs are hosts of many serious zoonoses. *See Irrigation, chapter 7,* for an example of JE associated with pig breeding and rice production.

The three most important zoonoses in the Sahel are anthrax, brucellosis and bovine tuberculosis. All are carried primarily by cattle. Brucellosis is a severe and incapacitating zoonotic disease important both where unpasteurised dairy products are consumed and as an occupational hazard of livestock and meat industries. Transmission is by direct contact between animals and man. Livestock movement is of particular concern. In areas where pastoralism is common many hospital patients who are treated for malaria or typhoid fever may actually have brucellosis. Random tests of patients in Karamoja, Uganda, revealed a prevalence of about 25%. A similar percentage of cattle herds were infected[1]. No information has been obtained regarding the importance of brucellosis in livestock development projects.

EXAMPLES

- After a human epidemic in the Cape Verde islands some 60% of animal sera were seropositive for Q Fever[5].

- In 1971 domestic pigs were imported into West New Guinea from a country in which cysticercosis (due to *Taenia solium*) was endemic in pigs and people. The parasite was absent from New Guinea. In 1974 there was an epidemic of severe burns among the Ekari people which was attributed to epileptic fits causing people to fall into fires. The fits were correlated with cerebral cysticercosis infection. The infection spread rapidly and was difficult to control due to husbandry practices and this is believed to have caused considerable economic loss[6,7].

- The present global distribution of cystic hydatid disease (due to *Echinococcus granulosus*) is associated with the widespread importation of sheep and dogs[8].

- Trichinosis in Africa is of rare human importance and caused by a strain of parasite which is not well adapted to domestic pigs. There is concern that new strains may be imported in domestic pigs from regions where it is of considerably greater importance[9].

Q Fever is emerging as a public health problem in areas of sheep, cattle rearing and dairy farms[2]. Human infection is usually through inhalation and abattoir workers are especially at risk[3,4].

1.2 NON-COMMUNICABLE DISEASE

Animal husbandry may entail exposure to a number of non-communicable diseases. These include asthma and allergic pneumonitis amongst those exposed to animal wastes, and occupational asthma, for example amongst those working with poultry. Noise may also be a substantial problem, for example amongst those working in chicken batteries.

1.3 MALNUTRITION

There is a general concern about the replacement of large areas of crop production by commercial livestock production. Livestock are inefficient at converting biomass to food compared with crops[10]. A unit of good agricultural land can support more people through the production of crops for human consumption than through livestock production. Often the direct nutritional benefits of commercial livestock production are not felt by the people in the producing areas. *See Agriculture, chapter 6, Choice of Crop.*

EXAMPLES

◆ In Mexico, livestock grain consumption changed from 6% to 50% between 1960 and 1985. In 1985, 25 million Mexicans were too poor to eat meat. The land planted to subsistence crops did not increase during the same period. The area planted for sorghum, a cattle feed, increased dramatically[11].

◆ During the 1960s, soybean became an important crop in Brazil. By the end of the 1970s it was the country's number one export – all going to feed Japanese and European livestock. At the same time the number of people suffering from hunger rose from one-third of the population in 1960 to two-thirds by the early 1980s[11].

In many parts of Africa women care for dairy cattle. Their investment of time and other resources has to be increased for supplying commercial dairies often at the expense of other food producing tasks. However, the dairies usually pay cash to the men. Women have increased their labour but lost an income source from occasional sales of milk and milk products[12]. The loss of cash income by women may lead to a reduction in family nutrition, as male priorities may be different. *See chapter 6, Agriculture, Choice of Crop.*

1.4   INJURY

In many rural societies in developing countries, livestock represent an important form of wealth. Caring for animals does, however, pose a number of potential injury hazards including animal bites, being gored by horns (eg. by goats and cows), lacerations, cuts and fractures from kicks, falls from animals and crush injuries.

2   DRUG RESIDUES

2.1   COMMUNICABLE DISEASE

In some countries large proportions of livestock receive drugs for therapy, prophylaxis or growth promotion. For example, chickens grow 10% faster when fed on antibiotics. Sub-therapeutic doses of antibiotic in the animal body and residues in the environment facilitate the development of resistant strains of bacteria, including *Salmonella*[13].

EXAMPLES

◆ A study in Alma Ata, Kazakhstan suggested that salmonella species isolated from poultry farm employees, shepherds, animals and fowls featured multiple antibiotic resistance, especially to the tetracycline family. This was possibly due to veterinary applications of antibiotics not only for treatment and prevention but also as food supplements[14].

◆ In the USA, an outbreak of salmonellosis resistant to many antibiotics was traced to hamburgers derived from antibiotic treated cattle[15].

2.2   NON-COMMUNICABLE DISEASE

When drugs are used in livestock the possibility exists that residues will occur in human food products. The parent drug is metabolised by the animal into many derivatives[16]. The maximum acceptable daily intake of either parent drug or derivatives has not always been established. Some of the drugs have known teratogenic potential.

EXAMPLES

◆ In Norway about twice as many antibiotics are consumed by animals and fish as by humans[13].

◆ In India about 80% of the animal production industry uses antibiotics and other drugs[17].

---

3 ANIMAL FEED CONTAMINATION

3.1 COMMUNICABLE DISEASE

Some 1500 million children under the age of five suffer from diarrhoea and 4–5 million die per year. Many diarrhoeal episodes may be due to foodborne rather than waterborne pathogens[18]. Some of these foodborne pathogens, such as *Listeria* and *Toxoplasma* are dangerous during pregnancy as infection of the foetus can cause death or serious malformations.

Animal feeds composed of meals partly of animal and partly of vegetable origin have shown to be contaminated with *Salmonella* and *Campylobacter*. Animals fed on such feeds in intensive breeding units shed large quantities of pathogens in their faeces that contaminate the wet surfaces of slaughter houses, meat processing and distribution plants. The large numbers of these carrier animals have contributed to the contamination of the environment and to the creation of infection cycles of foodborne diseases[18].

EXAMPLES

◆ In 1985 some 200,000 people were involved in an outbreak of salmonellosis in Chicago caused by consuming contaminated pasteurized milk[19].

◆ In 1989, the UK reported about 32,000 cases of Campylobacteriosis, a leading cause of foodborne disease[20].

3.2 NON-COMMUNICABLE DISEASE

The presence of residues of pesticides, herbicides, fumigants[21] and heavy metals[22] in livestock because of contaminated feeds is of potential health importance.

4 DAIRY FARMING

4.1 NON-COMMUNICABLE DISEASE

Dairy farming has been associated with increased prevalence of farmer's lung disease[23]. This is due to working long hours in enclosed spaces exposed to organic particulate matter.

EXAMPLE

◆ In the US, deaths due to farmer's lung disease are more common in the dairy industry than in other kinds of farming[23].

---

5   LIVESTOCK WASTES

5.1   COMMUNICABLE DISEASE

Livestock waste is increasingly discharged into rivers, rendering them hazardous as water sources. It is also used as fertilizer for field crops, vegetable gardens and fish ponds. Parasites are spread from the waste to people who handle fish and prepare or consume raw food. Slurry disbursed on land in hot climates aids the rapid growth of pathogens responsible for foot-and-mouth disease, tuberculosis and brucellosis.

Cryptosporidial infection is an emerging cause of diarrhoea among children and immuno-suppressed adults[24,25]. Contamination of drinking water with animal faecal matter is an important source of infection. Abattoir workers are also at risk.

Contact with poultry and an environment contaminated with animal faecal matter increases the transmission of *Salmonella* and *Campylobacter* to humans[26,27]. The wastewater discharges from poultry farms can carry heavy loads of these micro-organisms and may contaminate drinking water supplies[28].

EXAMPLES

◆ Abattoir workers in Holland associated with the pork industry have a 1500 times higher chance of getting meningitis associated with *Salmonella* infection than other workers[29].

◆ A study in Alma Ata, Kazakhstan, found that in industrial poultry farms, 16% of hens and 12% of ducks were infected with salmonella. The study established that humans develop the salmonella carrier state as a result of occupational exposure to poultry and rams[14].

5.2   NON-COMMUNICABLE DISEASE

Heavy metals in slurry are absorbed by vegetables and may be consumed by humans.

6   PASTORAL NOMADISM

See also Food Security and Agriculture, chapter 6.

USAID has published specific Guidelines for assessing the health impact of development projects in the Sahel[30]. See the table at the end of this chapter.

Nomadic pastoralists typically occupy the drier, poorer, more fragile and peripheral lands. They are often cut off from the political process and from access to important social infrastructure. Development projects often have the objective of sedentarization. They frequently fail, or cause irreversible environmental degradation. Provision of water supplies is often a priority.

EXAMPLE

◆ Most participants in dairy development projects in Kenya reserved insufficient milk to feed their children and sold the available milk for cash[31].

Nomadism has a sound ecological basis and the health of nomads is closely associated with the health of their environment.

6.1 COMMUNICABLE DISEASE

Commercial development of their lands pushes nomads into drier areas or denies them grass and water, increasing their marginalization. For example, more than 20,000 nomads were displaced from the Awash Valley in Ethiopia while 100,000 labourers and managers migrated from elsewhere to work on irrigated estates. The low population density and mobility of pastoralists often protect them and their livestock from some of the communicable diseases of settlement such as geohelminths and brucellosis[32]. Lack of water may intensify diseases with a direct faecal-oral route of transmission[33].

EXAMPLE

◆ The prevalence of hydatid disease among the Turkana in Kenya increases when they and their dogs are concentrated into camps during periods of drought[32].

Mothers and children are the most vulnerable component of nomadic communities. Small reductions in nutritional intake may impair their health and increase their susceptibility to communicable diseases[34].

Rainwater dams are often constructed for livestock watering. There is often conflict with domestic water requirements. Consequently, the dams provide foci of schistosomiasis transmission and a water supply contaminated with faecal matter.

In India and Nepal, particularly, there are huge populations of livestock which depend on forest forage as there is not enough grazing land[35]. Herders reside for considerable periods of the year in the forest where they contract malaria. As they circulate to their villages on the plains they disseminate the parasite.

TABLE I   Potential positive and negative effects on health of livestock development activities in the Sahel (modified from USAID[30]).

Activity	Positive effects	Negative effects
Animal health: vaccination programs, dipping tanks, disease control	Increased availability of high quality protein in the market area improving: human nutrition, animal health, marketability	Increased pressure on range resources, potential overgrazing, loss of ground cover Improper use of chemicals, concentration of toxic substances in water, soil, food
Livestock water supply	Increased herd size and number as water supply constraints ease, increased livestock survivorship. Improved animal health	Increased pressure on range resources (expanded potential for overgrazing and subsequent decline of soil fertility)
Pasture rehabilitation, restoration of vegetative cover	Increased carrying capacity of pastures Increased ecological stability. Improved soil fertility (water retention, nutrient content, decreased erosion)	Secondary effects of agricultural techniques employed to reseed and plough and increases in animal and human populations (exploitation of recovered land)
Relocation and resettlement of nomadic herders; herd management	Decrease in the number of herders and animals, protection of seasonal pastures from overgrazing. Fewer herds; fewer animals per herd; improved animal nutrition, increased market value; ecological stability of pasture, better water retention of soil, decreased erosion More marketable livestock, leading to improved cash flow, increased livestock sales, improved human nutrition	Increase in: population density in resettled areas; communicable diseases due to crowding and overuse of sanitation facilities; personal and ethnic conflict Lowered nutritional status: poor crop yields due to resettled people's unfamiliarity with farming methods; initial hunger due to impossibility of planting crops if resettled too late in growing season; unavailability of traditional foods, rejection of new foods due to unfamiliarity and ignorance of cooking methods; infantile malnutrition due to unfamiliarity with weaning foods; decreased farmland per capita in resettled areas

TABLE I   continued

Activity	Positive effects	Negative effects
Establishment of markets, slaughterhouses, storage and shipping facilities	Increased availability of high-quality protein in market area, improved nutrition, increased resistance to disease	Increase in zoonotic diseases due to meat processing: anthrax; brucellosis; bovine tuberculosis; cattle trypanosomiasis
	Attraction of merchants, more available cash, increased availability of commercial goods and services	Possible contamination of food and water supply
	Improved efficiency of livestock marketing	Overuse of sanitation facilities due to increased immigration: increase in food and water-borne diseases (dysenteries; typhoid, cholera, intestinal worms); increase in vector-borne diseases (malaria, schistosomiasis, trypanosomiasis)
	Decrease in livestock disease due to dipping in disinfectant	

6.2   NON-COMMUNICABLE DISEASE

Small-scale livestock development projects can provide a vehicle for improving mother and child care and introducing family planning programmes by gaining the confidence of the community[36]. The disadvantages of permanent settlement must be balanced against the better access to improved health services in settled communities.

6.3   MALNUTRITION

Boreholes can cause overgrazing. Human and livestock population densities can soon be raised above carrying capacity. Food security is determined by animal ownership and the fulfilment of social obligation through animal exchange. Environmental degradation reduces food security and the buffering mechanisms that enable the community to withstand droughts and other disasters.

7   REFERENCES

1   D G K Ndyabahinduka, and I H Chu, "Brucellosis in Uganda." *Int J Zoonoses.* 1984, 11:59–64.

2   G H Lang, "Q fever: an emerging public health concern in Canada." *Can J Vet Res.* 1989, 53:1:1–6.

3   R E Somma-Moreira, R M Caffarena, S Somma, G Perez, and M Monteiro, "Analysis of Q fever in Uruguay." *Rev Infect Dis.* 1987, 9:2:386–387.

4   L A Sawyer, D B Fishbein, and J E McDade, "Q fever: current concepts." *Rev Infect Dis.* 1987, 9:5:935–946.

5   W Sixl, and B Sixl-Voigt, "Research on a possible Q-fever infection in humans and animals on the Cape Verde Islands (Santa Cruz/Santiago, West Africa)." *J Hyg Epidemiol Microbiol Immunol.* 1987, 31:4 supplement:472–474.

6   D C Gajdusek, "Introduction of *Taenia solium* into West New Guinea with a note on an epidemic of burns from cysticercus epilepsy in the Ekari people of the Wissel Lakes area." *Papua New Guinea Med J.* 1978, 21:4:329–342.

7   S Gunawan, D B Subianto, and L R Tumada, "Taeniasis and cysticercosis in the Pania Lakes area of Irian Jaya." *Bulletin Penelitian Kesehaten Health Studies in Indonesia.* 1976, IV:1 & 2:9–17.

8   R C A Thompson, "Biology and speciation of *Echinococcus granulosus*." *Aust Vet J.* 1979, 55:March:93–98.

9   W C Campbell, "Trichinella in Africa and the *nelsoni* affair." in-*Parasitic Helminths and Zoonoses in Africa*, Ed. *C N L Macpherson and P S Craig.* (Unwin Hyman, London 1991).

10   D Pimental, and M Pimental, "Food, Energy and Society." *Resource and Environmental Sciences Series,* (Edward Arnold, London 1979).

11   F M Lappe, and J Collins, "World Hunger: 12 Myths." (Earthscan, London 1988).

12   Institutions and Agrarian Reform Division. FAO Food Policy and Nutrition Division and Human Resources, "Economic change and the outlook for nutrition." *Food and Nutr.* 1984, 10:1:71–79.

13 M Yndestad, "Public health aspects of residues in animal products: fundamental considerations." (1991) The Problems of Chemotherapy in Aquaculture. Office Internacional Epizooitology (unpublished).

14 A L Kotova, S A Kondratskaya, and I M Yasutis, "Salmonella carrier state and biological characteristics of the infectious agent." *J Hyg Epidemiol Microbiol Immunol.* 1988, 32:1:71–78.

15 G R Conway, and J N Pretty, "Unwelcome Harvest: Agriculture and Pollution." (Earthscan Publications, London 1991).

16 J P Cravedi, "Assessment of drug residues in fish: the role of metabolic studies." (1991) The Problems of Chemotherapy in Aquaculture. Office Internacional Epizooitology (unpublished).

17 Y P Singh, and V K Vijjan, "Ill effects associated with the use of feed additives in livestock production." *Livest Advis.* 1987, 12:11:33–36.

18 World Health Organization Commission on Health and Environment, "Report of the Panel on Food and Agriculture." (World Health Organization, Geneva 1992).

19 C A Ryan, M K Nickels, N T Hargrett-Bean, M E Potter, T Endo, L Mayer, C W Langkop, C Gibson, R C McDonald, and R T Kenney, "Massive outbreak of antimicrobial-resistant salmonellosis traced to pasteurized milk." *J Am Med Assoc.* 1987, 258:22:3269–3274.

20 UK Public Health Laboratory Services, "Communicable Disease Report." (December 1989) Public Health Laboratory Services, UK. 89/52.

21 M K Cordle, "USDA regulation of residues in meat and poultry products." *J Anim Sci.* 1988, 66:2:413–433.

22 K Vreman, N G van der Veen, E J van der Molen, and W G de Ruig, "Transfer of cadmium, lead, mercury and arsenic from feed into tissues of fattening bulls: chemical and pathological data." *Neth J Agric Sci.* 1988, 36:4:327–338.

23 D M Mannino, J E Parker, and M C Townsend, "Dairy farming production in the US and death with farmer's lung from 1976–1986: an ecological study." *Am Rev of Resp Dis Part 2.* 1990, 141:4:A588.

24 D F Wittenberg, E G Smith, J van den Ende, and P J Becker, "*Cryptosporidium*-associated diarrhoea in children." *Ann Trop Paediatr.* 1987, 7:113–117.

25 B A Rush, "*Cryptosporidium* and drinking water (Letter to the Editor)." *The Lancet.* 1987, 333:8559:632.

26 O Grados, N Bravo, R E Black, and J P Butzler, "Paediatric *Campylobacter* diarrhoea from household exposure to live chickens in Lima, Peru." *WHO Bull.* 1988, 66:3:369–374.

27 K Moelbak, N Hoejlyng, and K Gaarslev, "High prevalence of *Campylobacter* excreters among Liberian children related to environmental conditions." *Epidemiol Infect.* 1988, 100:2:227–237.

28 W Stelzer, H Mochmann, U Richter, and H J Dobberkau, "A study of *Campylobacter jejuni* and *Campylobacter coli* in a river system." *Zentralbl Hyg Umweltmed.* 1988, 189:1:20–28.

29 J P Arends, and H C Zanen, "Meningitis caused by *Streptococcus suis* in humans." *Rev Infect Dis.* 1988, 10:1:131–137.

30 Family Health Care Inc./USAID, "Health Impact Guidelines for the Design of Development Projects in the Sahel: Volume 1: Sector-Specific Reviews and Methodology." (13 April 1979) United States Agency for International Development, Washington. PN-AAJ-381.

31 A A J Jansen, H T Horelli, and V J Quinn, "Food and Nutrition in Kenya: A Historical Review." (University of Nairobi and UNICEF, Nairobi 1987).

32 D L Watson-Jones, and C N L Macpherson, "Hydatid disease in the Turkana district of Kenya: man:dog contact and its role in the transmission and control of hydatidosis amongst the Turkana." *Ann Trop Med Parasit.* 1988, 82:4:343–56.

33 H Kloos, G DeSole, and A Lemma, "Intestinal parasitism in semi-nomadic pastoralists and subsistence farmers in and around irrigation schemes in the Awash Valley, Ethiopia, with special emphasis on ecological and cultural associations." *Soc Sci Med.* 1981, 15(B):457–469.

34 Canadian International Development Agency, "Baseline Monitoring Phase of the FARM Camel Improvement Project." (1988) Canadian International Development Agency (unpublished).

35 A V Kondrashin, R K Jung, and J Akiyama, "Ecological aspects of forest malaria in Southeast Asia." in-*Forest Malaria in Southeast Asia, Proceedings of an Informal Consultative Meeting, WHO/MRC, 18–22 February 1991, Ed. VP Sharma and AV Kondrashin.* (World Health Organisation, New Delhi 1991).

36 B King, "Community-based Primary Health Care for Nomads in Association with Camel Livestock Development: A Family Approach." (AMREF, New York 1988).

chapter 11

PUBLIC SERVICE SECTOR HEALTH HAZARDS AND THE PROJECT STAGE AT WHICH SAFEGUARDS MAY BE REQUIRED

Urban Development

Project stage	Health hazard	Examples and causes
Location	Communicable Disease	Poor sanitation, water supply and food hygiene, overcrowding, displacement
	Non-Communicable Disease	Pollution, hazardous waste
	Injury	Steep hillsides, flood-prone valleys, poor access by emergency services
Planning and Design	Communicable Disease	Water supply and sanitation
	Non-Communicable Disease	Pollution
	Injury	Traffic
Construction	Communicable Disease	Poor sanitation, water supply and food hygiene, STDs, exposure to vectors
	Non-Communicable Disease	Inadequate occupational safety measures
	Injury	Inadequate occupational safety measures
Operation	Communicable Disease	Solid waste management, blocked drainage, domestic water storage
	Non-Communicable Disease	Substance abuse, stress
	Injury	Traffic, violence

Water Supply and Drainage

Project stage	Health hazard	Examples and causes
Location	Communicable Disease	Distance to domestic water supply, water contact diseases
Planning and Design	Communicable Disease	Inappropriate water supply and drainage systems
	Non-Communicable Disease	Pollution, mineral deficiency
Operation	Communicable Disease	Lack of health education, poor maintenance, poor protection, poor drainage

Refuse Disposal and Sanitation

Project stage	Health hazard	Examples and causes
Location	Communicable Disease	Contamination of groundwater by pathogens
	Non-Communicable Disease	Contamination of groundwater by chemicals
Planning and Design	Communicable Disease	Soil contamination by excreta, pit latrine design
Construction	Injury	Inadequate occupational safety
Operation	Communicable Disease	Creation of vector habitats by poor solid waste disposal
	Non-Communicable Disease	Air and water pollution, skin disorders
	Injury	Explosive gases, hand and leg injuries, lower back pain for refuse workers

Low Cost Housing

Project stage	Health hazard	Examples and causes
Location	Communicable Disease	Vector breeding sites
Planning and Design	Communicable Disease	Overcrowding, poor ventilation, poor wastewater disposal, domestic water supply
	Non-Communicable Disease	Smoke from cooking stoves
	Mental Disorder	Overcrowding, poor quality and noise, pollution resulting in anxiety, violence and substance abuse
Construction	Injury	Inadequate occupational safety
Operation	Injury	Structural failure, fire, falls

See also Transport and Communication, chapter 3, and "A review of Environmental Health Impacts in Developing Country Cities" [1].

There are many health hazards associated with the health sector that are outside the scope of this review. They include occupational health hazards of health workers such as infection, injury, poisoning and irradiation. Hospitals may have a negative impact on the surrounding environment and community through air and water pollution, hazardous solid wastes, increased traffic, increased cost of food in the local markets, poorly regulated supply and circulation of drugs.

1   URBAN DEVELOPMENT

'Very few governments or aid agencies give much attention to cities' environment problems — especially the problems that impact most on the health and livelihoods of poorer groups[2].'

Rapid urbanization is shifting the balance of population from rural to periurban environments throughout the world. In a few years, some 50% of the world population will be living in the 'septic fringe' of cities. This term includes a large range of housing types such as tenements, boarding houses, illegal sub-divisions and informal settlements[2]. Much of the population increase is due to natural change rather than in-migration.

The urban poor represent a vast and cheap labour supply. They participate actively in and are essential to the urban economy. Their well-being can ensure the stability of government[3].

1.1   COMMUNICABLE DISEASE

In the crowded conditions of urban slums there are epidemics of communicable disease, such as cholera and meningitis. Much infant mortality is due to diarrhoea exacerbated by malnutrition.

EXAMPLES

♦ Increased dust levels in poor areas coupled with overcrowding increases the risk of outbreaks of meningococcal meningitis[4,5,6].

♦ In Lagos and Manila some swamp and coastal lands were filled to form construction sites. In both cases the fill has blocked the waters of extensive river systems that sweep to the sea through wetlands. As a result large urban areas are now periodically flooded and water supplies contaminated[7].

♦ In Jakarta many people use private wells because of the lack of piped water. Unconstrained abstraction of groundwater has caused salt water to intrude into the aquifer in the northern part of the city and the shallow wells have become saline. Extensive development in the southern part of the city, combined with more distant deforestation and dumping of solid and liquid wastes into the rivers and canals that drain the city, has lead to increased runoff and heavy flooding in the north. Most of the city's poor live in the northern area and are debilitated by disease from the polluted floodwaters. To buy drinking water from vendor-drawn hand carts they must pay as much as 15 to 20 percent of their income, or twenty times the unit cost of piped water[7].

1.2   NON-COMMUNICABLE DISEASE

Urban development projects are usually concerned with water supply, sanitation, refuse collection, housing and roads. The most serious problems regarding impact on human health are due to government failures. There is frequently failure to control industrial pollution. City-dwellers are often denied the basic infrastructure and services essential for health[2].

EXAMPLES

◆ The river Ganges receives untreated sewage from 114 cities with populations of more than 50,000. Industries including DDT factories discharge untreated waste directly into the river[8].

◆ Untreated industrial and domestic effluents are discharged directly into lake Maryut in Egypt. Fish production has declined by 80% in the last decade[8].

The World Health Organization recommends the planning of effective systems of public transport to combat the growing pollution from fossil-fuelled transport[8].

EXAMPLE

◆ The annual average total particulate levels in Metro Manila range from 70–230 $\mu g/m^3$ and frequently exceed WHO guidelines[9].

Location and zoning is important for safeguarding health in the urban environment. Schools near to major highways may expose children to excess levels of traffic pollutants. Large distances between home and the workplace generate streams of pollution along commuter routes. Concentration of septic tanks at too high a density can affect the quality of drinking water.

Poor urban communities have very inadequate access to health care, especially when they are injured at work, fall ill from pollution or require emergency services.

1.3 INJURY

Communities built on steep slopes or waterlogged sites with narrow alleyways are inaccessible to ambulances and fire engines[2]. Fire, building collapse, landslide and wounds are frequent occurrences in such neighbourhoods[10]. Traffic related injuries are common where there is a poorly planned transport system, lack of public transport and heavy traffic on narrow streets.

1.4   MALNUTRITION

Official urban health statistics often fail to indicate that the health and nutritional status of the urban poor is worse than their rural counterparts.

Some 70% of households in urban slums are headed by women[11]. Young children must often be left unattended while their mother works. Childhood malnutrition is common and can be helped by provision of land for vegetable gardens, however small.

EXAMPLE

◆   In Manila owners of unused land were obliged to cultivate or forfeit it. Community gardens were established. One garden supplied 800 squatter families with 80% of their vegetables on 1500m^2 of land[3].

1.5   MENTAL DISORDER

Noise pollution at night leads to sleep disturbance. This may affect daytime performance, such as reaction times[8]. Background noise is a major problem in many cities. It could be reduced by good planning, legislation, education and engineering. Behavioural side-effects include anxiety and hostility.

Many physical characteristics of housing and the living environment have an influence on mental disorder and social pathology. Stressful factors include: noise, air, water or soil pollution, overcrowding, inappropriate design, inadequate maintenance of the physical structure and services, poor sanitation or a high concentration of specific toxic substances. Psychosocial health problems include: depression, drug and alcohol abuse, suicide, child and spouse abuse, delinquency, and target violence (eg. rape, teacher assault). It is increasingly recognised that environment influences violent behaviour and that the initiatives which help to combat infectious diseases could be used to combat violence. Strong social networks have beneficial effects on psychosocial problems, especially for children, and care should be taken that these are not disrupted when authorities plan rehousing.

2 WATER SUPPLY PROJECTS

2.1 COMMUNICABLE DISEASE

The communicable diseases associated with water are commonly subdivided as follows:

WATER WASHED

These diseases are prevented by washing and bathing.

WATER BORNE

These diseases are prevented by pathogen free water supply.

WATER BASED

Schistosomiasis and guinea worm (dracunculiasis) are important examples of diseases where the pathogen spends most of its life in water.

WATER RELATED

Many insect vectors, such as mosquitoes, require a special kind of water during their immature life stage.

Water supply projects often require the intermediate storage of domestic water in small containers and roof tanks. Small containers provide breeding places for *Aedes* mosquitoes that are vectors of dengue fever. Dengue is now widespread in urban areas of developing countries. Roof and ground level tanks in India and the Middle East provide breeding sites for a malaria mosquito which leads to widespread urban malaria. Leakage from water pipes and runoff from standpipe aprons provide additional mosquito breeding sites.

EXAMPLE

◆ As a result of a dengue epidemic in Bangkok in 1987, some 152,840 people required hospitalization at an estimated cost of $16M. The vector control budget for the same year is said to have been less than $300,000[12].

Safe drinking water supply projects are important for the eradication of guinea-worm which is a significant cause of morbidity in endemic areas[13]. Unfortunately, the wells that should help to prevent contamination are often poorly sited, badly built or break down.

EXAMPLES

◆ In Imo State, Nigeria, 58% of individuals infected with guinea-worm were unable to leave their compounds for a mean of 4.2 weeks. The absentee rate in schools rose to 60% during the transmission season[13].

◆ A village in Ho district, Ghana, had a hand pump for five years. The slight saltiness of the water deterred enough people to sustain guinea-worm infection from a more distant source[15].

Increased quantity of water is often more important than improved quality for the control of endemic diarrhoea[14]. Fetching and carrying water is often the role of women. Improved supply may provide extra time for child care and other activities.

Communities need convenient access to 30–50 litres of water per person per day. This must be accompanied by concurrent and continuing health education to have a health benefit. Sustainable water supplies require sustainable cultural changes. The cost of sustained water supplies should be borne largely by the community. Maintained protection of the source and distribution system is also essential. In the 1980s many water supply projects were planned and carried out on a 'top down' basis. The frequent result was unusable, costly installations as handpumps broke, treatment plants failed and communities were left with poor, if not worse, health conditions than before[8]. Piped water supplies usually leak and if the water pressure is low the leakage is inwards and the supply becomes heavily contaminated. Indiscriminate addition of extra taps reduces the pressure and increases the risk of contamination. Chlorination at source is not always effective[15].

EXAMPLES

◆ Access to public water is limited. In Bangkok and Jakarta about ⅓ of the community buy water from vendors. The price is five times that of piped water. In Pikine, Dakar, there are 696 persons per standpipe[2].

◆ A water supply project in Ethiopia was developed in collaboration with local women's groups. Its success was attributed to the high level of involvement of local communities and the development of maintenance and administration skills. Improved health and income generating projects were achieved[8].

A supply of clean water does not, in itself, ensure appropriate use or health improvement. Where groundwater is unpalatable due to excess salts, communities may use surface water contaminated with bacteria[16]. House clean-

EXAMPLES

◆ A study in Bangladesh concluded that water supply and sanitation hardware did not, in itself, reduce diarrhoea[17]. However, a study in Indonesia concluded that a piped water supply did significantly reduce the prevalence of conjunctivitis, skin and diarrhoea disease[18].

◆ A recent study investigated the relationship between diarrhoea and various risk factors in the Linggi river basin, Malaysia[19]. Water quality in the study area was constrained: the town sewage outfall was upstream of the town water supply intake; there was a lack of waste treatment by rubber processing plants and other industries; not all communities had access to piped water. The statistical significance of the results are indicated in the following table.

Risk factors in self-reporting diarrhoea, Malaysia[19].

Significance	Risk factors
High	Race, frequency of boiling water, type of toilet facility, sanitary water source, clean kitchen, clean children
Moderate	Treated water, drinking water source, yard free of garbage
Slight	Sink in house, sink in kitchen
Not significant	Crowding, village, town or estate, child carer, breast feeding, frequency of water shortage, indiscriminate defecation, flooding, children playing in dirt

The study concluded that while water supply and treatment were both important determinants of diarrhoea, other variables acted to minimise these determinants. Some of these variables were associated with location and others depended on human behaviour and education, as follows:

(i) Community vulnerability

The community consisted of several distinct cultural groups including Chinese, Indian, Malay and Orang Asli. Incidence rates were much higher in the Indian and Orang Asli communities. Behaviour varied between communities such as boiling of polluted water and cleaning children and kitchens.

(ii) Environmental factors

The most vulnerable communities did not have access to clean water and the design of their houses did not include a kitchen sink or a good toilet.

ing may be afforded higher priority than hand washing. Without prolonged and sustained health education there may be no changes in behaviour of the kind required to improve health. The 'software' of human education and behaviour is often more important than the engineering 'hardware'.

2.2   NON-COMMUNICABLE DISEASE

Underground supplies are generally well protected. The slow natural flow of water through earth, filters and kills pathogens. Mineral oils are the more serious pollutant, being long-lived, difficult to remove and tainting.

Minerals and trace elements in drinking water are natural and essential. The absence or excess of chemicals such as chlorides and fluorides affects health. Seasonal variation is common.

EXAMPLES

◆ Piped drinking water from a remote upland catchment increased goitre in one district of Malawi. It did not provide the iodine of the former, less clean, supply[20].

◆ In Kenya 61% of boreholes surveyed had excessive fluoride levels[21].

---

3   DRAINAGE

3.1   COMMUNICABLE DISEASE

Domestic water supplies are often installed before attention is given to providing adequate means for sullage water disposal. Single buckets from distant standpipes can be disposed to top soil. As water supply increases, specific methods of disposal must be planned to prevent surface pooling and contamination with sewage. Householders may then dig shallow soakpits or simply divert wastewater into the street. In areas with a high water table the accumulations of wastewater provide excellent breeding sites for mosquitoes that may transmit filariasis. Where waste or storm water is conducted through open drains, the drains are frequently blocked by solid refuse. Pooling of standpipe surrounds leads to contamination of shallow groundwater by water re-entry.

EXAMPLES

◆ In India there has been a rapid rise in lymphatic filariasis and the mosquito vector associated with the steady rise in the growth of human populations in endemic areas.

◆ *Anopheles stephensi*, the principal vector of urban malaria, has adapted to the urban environment in India and the Eastern Mediterranean. Some Anopheline mosquitoes now breed in ditches and swamps surrounding urban areas in Nigeria and Turkey[8].

Rainwater drains in tropical areas must be large to hold storm flows. They should be kept separate from either grey water or fouled sewage. Inadequate rainwater drainage in residential areas creates surface pooling. Drains should connect to culverts fitted with steel entry grills.

4 SANITATION PROJECTS

4.1 COMMUNICABLE DISEASE

Faecal-oral infections are those caused by pathogens in excreta reaching the mouth through food, water, hands, or air. The associated diseases reduce human productivity and kill children and the infirm. They range from a mild gastroenteritis to cholera and typhoid. The associated diseases are major causes of morbidity, mortality and hospital admission in developing countries. Women and children often benefit more than men by reductions in diarrhoea associated with improved water supply and excreta disposal. Soil contaminated by human excreta can result in worm infestations, such as hookworm. Symptoms include anaemia and blood loss.

EXAMPLES

◆ An epidemic of El Tor cholera in the densely populated and poorly served suburbs of Lusaka caused high mortality during 1990/91/92[20].

◆ In Dakar, nearly 1/6 of human faeces are dumped outside proper toilet facilities[22].

◆ In Dar es Salaam, 89% of households have only simple pit latrines. Many overflow during the wet season[2].

◆ A survey in Manila of 238 slum children found 92% with whipworm, 80% with roundworm and 10% with hookworm. 84% had at least two species of parasite[8].

While faecal matter decays rapidly, the pathogens which it contains survive for longer periods and even multiply. Modern sewage disposal systems usually fail to kill pathogens sufficiently. Viable pathogens remain in sludge and final effluent unless a disinfecting tertiary treatment is included. The use of waste stabilization ponds is the only waterborne sewage disposal system which approaches total pathogen destruction.

Water closets and bucket latrines do not dispose of waste, they merely store it for disposal elsewhere.

Underground disposal via pit latrine or soakaway uses the earth as a treatment process. The earth is an excellent processor of excreta. Pathogens are contained within 10m and chemical decomposition is complete within 20m. The capacity of the earth can be overwhelmed by excessive loading and high human densities. Shallow wells may become contaminated by nitrates.

Effective sewage systems are rare or absent in most urban centres, serving only the rich, the commercial centres and government offices[2]. Outbreaks of diarrhoea are often seasonal and associated with rainfall or high temperature[23].

Lack of suitable drainage of wastewater can saturate some soils causing disastrous mudslides. Examples are in squatter settlements of Rio de Janiero and Mameyes in Puerto Rico[15].

Family latrines are more effective than communal latrines because of maintenance and cleanliness problems. However, the cost of a septic tank falls rapidly when it serves 10–20 households[24]. Poor siting, design and maintenance of septic tanks reduce retention times, releasing pathogen rich effluent to contaminate groundwater. Sanitation projects can have a large impact on soil helminths and tapeworms. Improved personal hygiene can have a large impact on faecal-oral infections[16]. Washing facilities should be included. Septic tanks should be well sealed to prevent mosquito and fly breeding. An efficient ground irrigation disposal system is essential.

Public latrines require continuous servicing and must have a more durable construction. They may serve only the traditional owners of the land on which they are sited.

EXAMPLES

◆ A public latrine in a Ghanaian village was used by only 10% of a population of 2,000, despite its convenience and good quality[15].

Construction of pit latrines can often encourage the breeding of mosquitoes that transmit filariasis. Simple methods of prevention are available. The problem is particularly acute where there is a high water table.

EXAMPLE

◆ Polystyrene balls poured on wet pit latrines form an effective barrier against mosquito breeding. The reduction in infectious bites per person can be greater than 99.7%[25].

---

5 REFUSE DISPOSAL

Infrequent collection and rapid decomposition of wastes provide an attractive feeding and breeding site for flies, rats and other scavengers. Human and animal faecal matter or hospital wastes are often mixed with the refuse. Vectors and pathogens multiply. Domestic, and on occasion industrial, solid wastes are disposed of in open spaces within residential areas[8].

Collection and disposal of refuse can consume up to 50% of a municipal operating budget. In many otherwise good systems, only 50–70% of the refuse is regularly collected. The problem is organizational rather than technical. Refuse disposal is often a non-profit making business and thus is treated as an unwanted side-effect of development. Attention should be paid to storage, collection, transport, intermediate transfer to bulk transport and final disposal.

In some regions waste recovery is an important private industry employing many thousands of scavengers who may live or work on refuse dumps. They are referred to as human scavengers or waste pickers and are frequently ignored in urban project plans although their activities may be vital to the life of the city. Many consist of abandoned children and destitute families. They live and work under extensive health risks, which are largely undocumented, and suffer severe exploitation and deprivation. Suggested health hazards include raised levels of infant mortality, hand and leg injuries, intestinal and respiratory infections, eye infections, lower back pain, malnutrition, skin disorders and exposure to hazardous waste[26,27]. Water supply, for drinking and washing, and sanitation facilities are usually very poor at dump sites. Health and welfare facilities are required.

EXAMPLES

◆ Mexico City has 10,000 scavengers of the city dump. Cairo has 16,000 traditional refuse collectors who recycle nearly half of the 5,000 tonnes of daily waste[28].

◆ The total number of people in Asian cities whose occupation consists of waste recovery and recycling is believed to be several million and growing[26,29]. Some 1–2% of the urban population may be so employed.

◆ More than 14,000 people are said to live and work on "Smokey Mountain", one of Manila's dumpsites. Jakarta may have over 12,000 waste pickers. More than 40,000 people may gain their livelihood from waste in Calcutta[26].

Waste pickers may make a substantial contribution to urban waste management. They may reduce the volume of waste by 10–20%. However, private collection at source may only operate in the wealthy areas where refuse contains items of value. Observers agree that the issue of waste pickers cannot be evaded. Their positive role in the management of urban solid waste should be recognised and their lot improved[29]. Legislation against waste pickers is no solution.

5.1   COMMUNICABLE DISEASE

Houseflies may be important in the transmission of enteric infections, particularly those responsible for infantile diarrhoea and dysenteries.

Disease transmission by houseflies is greatest where inadequate refuse storage, collection and disposal (leading to increased breeding) is accompanied by inadequate sanitation. Thus flies gain greater access to human faeces. Refuse must be collected twice per week to prevent fly breeding.

EXAMPLES

◆ The role of houseflies in disease transmission has been shown by instances in Palestinian refugee camps, where the breakdown of chemical control has led to dramatic increases in infantile diarrhoea[30,31].

◆ Experimental trials using chemical control methods in Texas and Georgia demonstrated that diarrhoea attack rates may be up to 33% higher when houseflies are uncontrolled. Prevalence of the dysentery organism *shigella* was three-fold higher in untreated areas whilst death rates from diarrhoea and dysentery were measurably greater where houseflies remained uncontrolled[32,33].

Domestic rats, birds and other scavenging animals act as reservoirs for many organisms transmissible to people, including plague, forms of typhus, leptospirosis, trichinosis, psittacosis and salmonella infection.

Chemical control of both houseflies and rodents is not very effective because of widespread resistance. The essential basis of control remains denial of access to food and harbourage, by covered storage and efficient removal.

Aedes mosquitoes, vectors of dengue and yellow fever, breed prolifically in discarded containers that trap rainwater. *Culex* mosquitoes, vectors of filariasis, breed in polluted stagnant water. Such breeding sites often occur where drains are blocked by solid waste.

5.2   NON-COMMUNICABLE DISEASE

Once collected in poorly designed or poorly operated disposal sites, rubbish may contaminate groundwater with nitrates, heavy metals and other chemicals. Incineration of wastes may pollute the air with particulates and oxides of sulphur and nitrogen. The slag and ashes from incinerators may result in leachates that are rich in heavy metals and other potentially toxic substances[34].

5.3   INJURY

Combustible gases will be generated from waste tips for more than 20 years and these travel under roads and through ducts to create a hazard in buildings.

People collecting rubbish may be injured by sharp objects including glass, metal and wood. These may lead to puncture wounds and lacerations which may become infected and cause serious morbidity. Composted solid waste can cause injury to farmers as sharp objects are not always properly removed[36].

EXAMPLE

◆   Turkey, April 1993, methane from a rubbish tip exploded killing at least 13, injuring 100 and destroying homes[35].

---

6   LOW COST HOUSING

The linkage between housing and health is widely recognised but hard to evaluate. Important features are:

◆   protective structure;
◆   provision of water supplies;

◆   waste disposal facilities;

◆   structural safety of the site;

◆   overcrowding especially causing unintentional injuries and air-borne infection;

◆   indoor air pollution from domestic fuel;

◆   safe food storage;

◆   disease vectors;

◆   safety of equipment and chemicals used in home industry;

◆   psycho-social factors.

In most countries, the health authorities have not taken much part in urban planning[11]. Little, if any, attention by architects and planners is paid to the need for disease control and public health programmes[2]. Measures to provide housing for the urban poor include site and services programmes and slum upgrading programmes. These programmes often meet with mixed success because of their complex administrative requirements. On the one hand they legalise the occupation of land creating a sense of permanency in which infrastructure and services can develop. On the other hand, inflexible regulatory and standard-setting measures, designed to promote a safe and healthy housing environment, may be unaffordable. They may actually inhibit improvements in sanitation or in extension of services.

EXAMPLES

◆ Globally some 600 million urban dwellers and more than 1000 million rural inhabitants live in hazardous housing. These are characterized by overcrowding and lack of basic services such as piped water, sanitation and health care[8].

◆ 30%–60% of urban populations live in illegal settlements or in over-crowded tenements[8].

Public housing projects often concentrate scarce resources on relatively few units. They often benefit wealthier groups. More widely targeted infrastructure projects have adversely affected health due to displacement, or lack of community participation, or lack of health promoting features[8].

6.1   COMMUNICABLE DISEASE

House design and improvement has an important role in the control of vector-borne diseases such as malaria and Chagas' disease[37]. Poor design in low cost housing schemes can lead to the proliferation of vector-borne diseases. The most common problems arise either through inadequate provision for wastewater disposal or through construction on land with a high water table. Lack of storm water drainage can reduce ground stability and increase the sense of insecurity. Low construction costs can be associated with high maintenance costs; the objective should be to reduce both.

EXAMPLE

◆ Insecticidal paints developed in Brazil not only improve the appearance of rooms but also protect them from infestation by bugs that transmit Chagas' disease[38].

Environmental management is important in the control of disease vectors in and around homes and in lessening the risk of human infection. Important factors include:

◆ location of housing (eg. away from water which breeds mosquitoes);

◆ restricting the vectors' access to humans (eg. bed screens);

◆ restricting the vectors' food sources or breeding sites (eg. storage of food, removal of wastes);

◆ restriction of hiding places (cracks and dark areas)[8].

There is a high level of air-borne infection in people who live in over-crowded dwellings. Acute respiratory infections, tuberculosis, pneumonia, influenza and meningitis are all common. Poor nutrition, lack of health care, and a high percentage of children increase the infection rate[8].

EXAMPLES

◆ The cost of TB immunization is less than US$6 per person. The cost of treatment is US$30–50 per person[8].

◆ The City Corporation of Yangon (Rangoon) built low-cost satellite towns on reclaimed swampy land to accommodate large numbers of squatters. Although protected from flooding by bunds and sluice gates, the ground became waterlogged during the rains. The surface drains were inadequate, mosquitoes bred heavily, and Bancroftian filariasis transmission was soon established[39].

◆ Multi-storied blocks of flats were also constructed with good internal plumbing but not connected to the city sewage system. Pools of polluted waste water were formed and mosquitoes proliferated[39].

◆ Outbreaks of leptospirosis in Sao Paulo and Rio de Janeiro are associated with flooding, high population density, presence of rats, cats and dogs and proximity to waste tips[8].

6.2   NON-COMMUNICABLE DISEASE

Adequate ventilation of housing is essential for good health. This should include two series of vents permitting cross ventilation to all parts of the building. A recent review of domestic biofuel and health, notes that women and children spend prolonged periods in unventilated houses exposed to smoke from cooking stoves. See Energy, chapter 5, Biomass Fuels.

6.3   INJURY

The health problems linked to unsafe or dangerous building structures include increased risk of fire, building collapse and electrocution. Many shelters are built of highly flammable materials. Open cooking fires, candles, burning of wastes and close proximity of neighbours increase the fire risk. Injuries from falls are common. The elderly and young children are most vulnerable. Lack of parental care due to working away from home is an associated factor[8].

EXAMPLE

◆   A survey of 599 slum children in Rio de Janeiro found that unintentional injuries accounted for 19% of all health problems of which 66% were falls, 17% cuts and 10% burns[8].

Poor urban developments may be associated with an increased risk of violent crime. Violence directed against women, both physical and sexual, may increase in such environments and are exacerbated by ready availability of alcohol. Lack of street-lighting, overcrowded households and poor public policing systems may increase the risks of violence.

7   REFERENCES

1 D Bradley, C Stephens, T Harpham, and S Cairncross, "A Review of Environmental Health Impacts in Developing Country Cities." Discussion Paper 6 (World Bank Urban Management Programme, 1992).
2 J E Hardoy, and D Satterthwaite, "Environmental problems of third world cities – a global issue ignored?" Public Admin and Dev. 1991, 11:4:341–361.
3 T Harpham, T Lusty, and P Vaughan, "In the Shadow of the City." (Oxford University Press, Oxford 1987).
4 B Schwartz, P S Moore, and C V Broome, "Global epidemiology of meningococcal disease." Clin Microbiol Rev. 1989, 4:2 supplement:S118–124.
5 M A Salih, H S Ahmed, Z A Karrar, I Kamil, K A Osman, Palmgren H, Y Hofvander, and P Olcen, "Features of a large epidemic of group A meningococcal meningitis in Khartoum, Sudan." Scand J Infect Dis. 1988, 22:2:161–170.

6 P S Moore, L H Harrison, E E Telzak, G W Ajello, and C V Broome, "Group A meningococcal carriage in travellers returning from Saudi Arabia." *J Am Med Assoc.* 1988, 260:18:2686–2689.

7 J A Lee, "The Environment, Public Health and Human Ecology: Considerations for Economic Development." (John Hopkins University Press, Baltimore 1985).

8 World Health Organization Commission on Health and Environment, "Our Planet, Our Health." (World Health Organization, Geneva 1992).

9 R D Subida, and E B Torres, "Epidemiology of Chronic Respiratory Symptoms and Illnesses Among Jeepney Drivers, Air-conditioned Bus Drivers and Commuters Exposed to Vehicular Emissions in Metro Manila, 1990–1991." (November 1991) World Health Organization.

10 G Goldstein, "Life saving services." in-*The Poor Die Young: Housing and Health in Third World Cities, Ed. J E Hardoy, S Cairncross and D Satterthwaite.* (Earthscan Publications, London 1990).

11 D E C Cooper Weil, A P Alicbusan, J F Wilson, M R Reich, and D J Bradley, "The Impact of Development Policies on Health: A Review of the Literature." (World Health Organization, Geneva 1990).

12 K Ungchusak, and P Kunasol, "Dengue haemorrhagic fever in Thailand, 1987." *Southeast Asian J Trop Med Public Health.* 1988, 19:3:487–490.

13 R Muller, "Dracunculus in Africa." in-*Parasitic Helminths and Zoonoses in Africa, Ed. C N L Macpherson and P S Craig.* (Unwin Hyman, London 1991).

14 S Cairncross, "Water supply and the urban poor." in-*The Poor Die Young: Housing and Health in Third World Cities, Ed. J E Hardoy, S Cairncross and D Satterthwaite.* (Earthscan Publications, London 1990).

15 E Potts, Personal observation.

16 S Cairncross, and R G Feachem, "Environmental Health Engineering in the Tropics: An Introductory Text." (John Wiley & Sons, Chichester 1983).

17 F J Henry, Y Huttly, Y Patwary, and K M Aziz, "Environmental sanitation, food and water contamination and diarrhoea in rural Bangladesh." *Epidemiol Infect.* 1990, 104:2:253–259.

18 S Wasito, S S Soesanto, and I B I Gotamo, "The health impact of drinking water supply in rural district of Sumedang, West Java." *Penelitan Kesehatan Buletin, Republik Indonesia.* 1989, 16:4:6–11.

19 S Lonergan, and T Vansickle, "Relationship between water quality and human health: a case study of the Linggi river basin in Malaysia." *Soc Sci Med.* 1991, 33:8:937–946.

20 E Potts, Personal communication.

21 K R Nair, F Manji, and J N Gitonga, "The occurrence and distribution of fluoride in groundwaters of Kenya." (1984) D E Walling, S S D Foster and P Wurzel Ed., Challengers in African Hydrology and Water Resources. Harare, Zimbabwe. International Association of Hydrological Sciences Publications, Washington DC.

22 S Cairncross, J E Hardoy, and D Satterthwaite, "The urban context." in-*The Poor Die Young: Housing and Health in Third World Cities, Ed. J E Hardoy, S Cairncross and D Sattherthwaite.* (Earthscan Publications, London 1990).

23 R H Meakins, "The role of health and environment in development with specific reference to Southern Africa." in-*Southern Africa Research for Development, Ed. M M Sefali.* (ISAS, NUL, Roma, Lesotho 1988).

24 G Sinnatamby, "Low cost sanitation." in-*The Poor Die Young: Housing and*

PUBLIC SERVICES

Health in Third World Cities, Ed. J E Hardoy, S Cairncross and D Satterthwaite. (Earthscan Publications, London 1990).

25 C A Maxwell, C F Curtis, Hamadi Haji, Shaban Kisumku, Abdul Issa Thalib, and Salum Ali Yahya, "Control of Bancroftian filariasis by integrating therapy with vector control using polystyrene beads in wet pit latrines." *Trans R Soc Trop Med Hyg.* 1990, 84:5:709–714.

26 A Z Bubel, "Waste picking and solid waste management." *Envir San Rev.* 1990, 30:53–66.

27 B L Adan, V P Cruz, M Palaypay, and G J Trezek, "Scavenging in Metro Manila." (March 1982) The Metro Manila Solid Waste Management Study. Task 11.

28 L Jensen, "Sorting out solutions to waste." *Source UNDP.* 1990, 2:2:13.

29 C Furedy, "Social aspects of solid waste recovery in Asian cities." *Envir San Rev.* 1990, 30:1–52.

30 L S West, "Fly Control in the Eastern Mediterranean and Elsewhere; Report of a Survey and Study." (12 May 1953) World Health Organisation. WHO/Insecticides/19.

31 J Keiding, "Report on a Consultancy on Control of House Flies and Other Insects of Public Health Importance in the Eastern Mediterranean Region." (31 March–9 May 1964) World Health Organisation.

32 J Watt, and D R Lindsay, "Diarrheal disease control studies 1. Effect of fly control in a high morbidity area." *Public Health Rep.* 1948, 63:41:1319–1334.

33 D R Lindsay, W H Stewart, and J Watt, "Effect of fly control on diarrhoeal disease in an area of moderate morbidity." *Public Health Rep.* 1953, 68:4:361–367.

34 World Health Organization, "Environmental Pollution Control in Relation to Development." (1985) World Health Organization. Technical Report Series No. 718.

35 Associated Press, "Refuse kills 13." *The Times.* London, 1993; Thursday, April 29th:15.

36 D Nicolaisen, U Plog, E Spreen, and S B Thapa, "Solid Waste Management with People's Participation. An Example in Nepal." (GTZ, Eschborn 1988).

37 C J Schofield, R Briceno-Leon, N Kolstrup, D J T Webb, and G B White, "The role of house design in limiting vector-borne disease." in-*The Poor Die Young: Housing and Health in Third World Cities*, Ed. J E Hardoy, S Cairncross and D Satterthwaite. (Earthscan Publications, London 1990).

38 L A Lacey, A D Alessandro, and M Barreto, "Evaluation of a chlorpyrifos-based paint for the control of triatominae." *Bull Soc Vector Ecol.* 1989, 14:1:81–86.

39 W W Macdonald, "Control of *Culex quinquefasciatus* in Myanmar (Burma) and India: 1960–1990." *Ann Trop Med Parasit.* 1991, 85:165–172.

chapter 12

MANUFACTURE AND TRADE SECTOR HEALTH HAZARDS AND THE PROJECT STAGE AT WHICH SAFEGUARDS MAY BE REQUIRED

Project stage	Health hazard	Examples and causes
Location	Communicable Disease	Contact with endemic disease foci
	Non-Communicable Disease	Pollution
	Malnutrition	Loss of common property resources
	Injury	Explosion and fire
Planning and Design	Non-Communicable Disease	Pollution, hazardous waste
	Injury	Work place design
Construction	Communicable Disease	Poor sanitation, water supply and food hygiene, STDs, exposure to vectors
	Non-Communicable Disease	Inadequate occupational safety measures
	Injury	Inadequate occupational safety measures
Operation	Communicable Disease	Zoonoses, STDs
	Non-Communicable Disease	Respiratory disease, miscarriage, foetal damage, cancer due to poor occupational safety and pollution, substance abuse, food contamination, skin disease
	Malnutrition	Market distortion, loss of common property resources
	Injury	Occupational safety, traffic, child labour
	Mental Disorder	Increased pace and monotonous nature of work resulting in stress, ill health and absenteeism

1   INTRODUCTION

Industrial activity affects the health of two vulnerable groups: the work force, through occupational safety and health; and the general population, through industrial pollution. In addition, catastrophic incidents can affect both groups. There are several recent reviews[1,2,3]. Health hazards include not only those of the production process but also those of raw materials, fuels, and wastes as they are obtained, transported and handled, and the effects on health of the products and wastes[4]. Related issues include: siting and zoning, control of industrial pollution, management of hazardous waste, disaster preparedness, and urbanization.

There are many important policy issues that are outside the scope of this review. These include: the establishment of 'pollution havens', the export of hazardous processes from developed to developing nations; the deliberate under-assessment of hazards and flouting of regulations; and the inability of governments to monitor and enforce. Many governments lack the resources for adequate risk assessment and risk management.

EXAMPLES

◆   At Koko, a Nigerian seaport, a large number of dumped chemical drums were found: these contained volatile solvents that with fire or explosions could produce highly toxic gases. Many of the drums, exported from Italy in 1987 and 1988, were damaged and leaking or were swelling from the heat[5].

◆   The increased regulation of the asbestos industry in many developed nations has caused multinationals to move production to developing nations. One such plant was described in 1981 in which the work-force were not protected from asbestos fibre[3].

There is a widespread, but probably mistaken, belief that environmental protection can only be achieved at the expense of economic growth.

2   INDUSTRIAL POLLUTION

Industrial pollution of air and water may be due to routine or unintentional discharge. The health risk is determined by the nature and amount of emission, local geography, climate and community location.

2.1   NON-COMMUNICABLE DISEASE

Unintentional discharges of acute poisons can occur when plants malfunction. The primary safeguard is proper plant maintenance and operation, including containment procedures, trained staff and emergency response plans. Additional safeguards include land zoning policy based on the known area of fallout of toxic emissions. Unfortunately, the potentially hazardous land around chemical plants is often settled by the urban poor. Enforcement of land zoning legislation, where it exists, is difficult. Foreign exchange restrictions often limit the availability of spare parts. Unintentional release also occurs during transport, storage or as a result of fires and collisions[4].

EXAMPLE

◆ The unintentional release of methyl isocyanate at Bhopal, India, led to over 6,000 deaths and many more injuries. Settlement of land adjoining the plant was an important factor contributing to the magnitude of the disaster. There is evidence that lower operating standards were employed than the norm[6].

Normal discharge of atmospheric pollution in urban areas is so high that 70% of populations may be living in areas where air quality conditions are unacceptable[1,7,8]. Threshold risk levels vary with climate, altitude, nutrition and infections. The families of workers may be exposed to hazardous materials such as lead and asbestos brought home on workers' clothing or by visiting the workplace. Young children are particularly susceptible[4].

EXAMPLES

◆ Respiratory ill-health in Sao Paulo, Brazil, is significantly associated with pollution levels. Poor socio-economic conditions aggravate the problem[7].

◆ Proximity of residential neighbourhoods to USA chemical plants was significantly associated with respiratory complaints in school children[8].

◆ In Utah, USA, changes in air-borne particulates associated with the closure and reopening of a steel mill between 1985 and 1988 was strongly correlated with hospital admission rates for various respiratory diseases[9].

Industrial waste is often released into water bodies that serve as water sources for large populations. In addition, fish stocks may become heavily polluted with heavy metals and other chemicals affecting fishers and consumers.

MANUFACTURE AND TRADE

EXAMPLES

◆ During the 1950's, the discharge of mercury into Minamata Bay, Japan, poisoned fish stocks and led to over 2,000 cases of serious neurological disease[10].

◆ Large reductions in fish catches as a result of pollution have been reported in Malaysia, Lake Maryut in Egypt, in the bay of Dakar and around the Indus delta near Karachi[4].

◆ The Kalu river flowing through Bombay's industrial suburbs is polluted by heavy metals from over 150 industrial units. Toxins, especially mercury and lead, are concentrated in the food chain affecting people in downstream villages[4].

◆ High concentrations of mercury, copper and cadmium have been found in fish from the south east Pacific coast of Latin America[4].

◆ In Brazil, mercury is widely used to remove impurities from gold and the discharge of wastes into rivers has led to contamination of the food chain posing a hazard to fish eating populations[4].

National agencies are nearly always inadequate for regulating discharges. Factories are relocated from industrialized to industrializing nations to evade legislation. Industrial activities tend to be concentrated in areas where there is already a concentration of commercial activity, including supply markets, communications technology and transport. Lack of land zonation brings vulnerable communities into contact with hazardous emissions and hazardous processes into contact with each other.

The cost of producing synthetic chemicals is sometimes less than the cost of their ultimate safe disposal. There is rarely adequate provision for the disposal of hazardous waste. A 'cradle-to-grave' approach has been advocated that encompasses generation, reduction, treatment, recovery, transport and disposal.

Most toxic waste is produced by the chemical industry. Other industries which produce significant amounts include the metal, petroleum, transport, electrical equipment, leather and tanning industries. Hospital wastes and sewage sludge are also considered hazardous[4].

EXAMPLES

◆ The industrial district of Cubato, Brazil, has 23 major industrial
plants and many smaller operations. Serious health problems include
elevated neonatal mortality rates, birth deformities, and a high prevalence of respiratory disorders. These are associated with high
levels of water and air pollution[11,12,13].

◆ Up to 1985, Mexico had no regulations governing disposal of the
16.5 million tonnes of hazardous waste that were generated each year[1].

◆ A study in China found dangerous levels of cadmium from a tungsten
ore dressing plant in irrigation water. The community was ingesting
the cadmium through agricultural crops. The average intake was
367–382 μgms per day. Many of the community had attributable
clinical symptoms[14].

2.2 INJURY

Industrial waste also carries a significant risk of injury. Injuries could occur
through fire, explosion, drowning, falls or inappropriate disposal of sharp
materials.

EXAMPLE

◆ At Guadalajara, Mexico, April 1992, a 2km length of sewer contaminated with alkines (such as petrol) exploded, killing more than
200 and injuring more than 800 people (International press).

---

3 OCCUPATIONAL HEALTH HAZARDS OF INDUSTRY

3.1 NON-COMMUNICABLE DISEASE AND INJURY

See also Mining, chapter 4 and Cross-Cutting Issues, chapter 2, Construction.

Occupational safety and health is too large and complex a subject to be
covered adequately in a broad review. It requires specialist treatment. There
is widespread agreement that little information is available from developing
countries. There is a recent review in "Proceedings of the International
Symposium on Health Impact of Rapid Industrialization and Urbanization
in Asia and the Pacific and its Public Health Activities"[15].

EXAMPLE

◆ Estimates suggest that globally there are 32.7 million occupational injuries per year and 146,000 deaths[4].

Three standard rates are used as indicators of occupational injury.

$$\text{Frequency rate} = \frac{number\ of\ disabling\ injuries}{employee\ hours\ of\ exposure} \times 1,000,000$$

$$\text{Severity rate} = \frac{total\ days\ charged}{employee\ hours\ of\ exposure} \times 1,000$$

Death rate = number of deaths per 1,000 workers

A wide range of health problems has been associated with industrial processes in industrialized nations. Ship builders in Italy, for example, have a high prevalence of respiratory disorders due partly to inhaling welding fumes[16]. Similar problems occur in developing nations but with poorer control and documentation[1]. Priorities are rarely established, for example pollution by pesticide may receive undue emphasis. Exposure limits are often modelled on those of developed countries and may be inappropriate because they do not take account of the different climate, nutritional status, genetic predisposition, work schedules and exposure levels. Where occupational health standards (OHS) are implemented, the larger industries are likely to receive the attention. Responsibility for OHS is often divided between many agencies. These may include the labour department, ministry of industry, environmental protection agency and ministry of public health.

EXAMPLES

◆ Extraction of scrap lead from car batteries is an important small industry. A Nairobi study noted that one third of the workforce tested had chronic lead poisoning. Lead dust levels in some enterprises were 1,000 times above threshold limit values. Face masks and protective clothing were often not provided or not properly used[17].

◆ Thailand is industrializing rapidly and had over 10,000 factories in 1988. Industrial injury claims have doubled in the last 10 years. Injuries and poisonings of all kinds were the second leading cause of adult mortality in 1985. There is a single centre for toxicology producing far fewer graduates per year than are needed[18].

Occupational diseases are regularly under-reported in some countries to avoid costly preventive measures. The annual rate of injuries to workers causing disablement is 21–34% in developing countries, compared with 3% in the UK during the 1970's[19]. A study by the Zimbabwe Congress of Trade Unions has suggested that reports of occupational injuries and diseases are only about 10% of what might be expected given the size of the workforce and rates experienced in Europe (where safety measures are more stringently applied)[20].

EXAMPLES

◆ Clubbing of the fingers and toes is a sign of chronic hypoxia. The symptoms were noted in match factory workers in Fiji exposed to Rhodamine B dye. The affected individuals did not use gloves or shower after work[21].

◆ Occupational health and safety is well developed in Singapore[22]. There are 1.25M workers in over 10,000 factories. Associated medical staff include: 260 physicians, 200 nurses, 10 industrial hygienists and 230 safety officers. The commonest recorded diseases are noise-induced deafness and dermatitis. The average frequency rate is 4. In the ship-building industry it is 14.

◆ A survey of silica dust-induced lung disease in the Philippines sampled workers in mining, ceramics, glass manufacturing and cement establishments. Using International Labour Organisation classifications, some 12% of the workers had small opacities[23]. This indicated the presence of silicosis which is not usually a disabling condition. It is, however, associated with an increased risk of tuberculosis.

The majority of the workforce may be engaged in small-scale industries with distinct occupational hazards that are not amenable to regulation or inspection. Child labour is a continuing and growing problem. A survey indicated that workers in small industries have a greater risk of suffering from toxic effects, or from fully developed occupational disease, than those in large industries[19].

EXAMPLE

◆ Over 50 deaths were documented due to leukaemia and bone marrow destruction in Turkish workers who used a glue based on benzene. The glue was introduced around 1965 and was cheaper than previously used substances. It was extensively used in the small shops of the leather industry. An active industrial hygiene or worker surveillance of small industries could have identified the problem, saved many lives and reduced the long term leukaemia risk for an estimated 28,000 Istanbul leather workers, as well as other workers in undocumented situations[4].

Noise-induced hearing loss is an increasing problem of industrialization and urbanization. Besides factories, the problem occurs in mining, forestry and transportation. Excessive noise interferes with communication, disrupts sleep, diminishes job performance and has other psychological effects[4]. Exposure to excessive noise levels above 90dBA for periods of greater than 10–15 years can lead to permanent hearing loss of the frequencies used in speech. Extremely high noise levels above 145dBA peak, such as produced by explosions or gun fire, can lead to immediate severe and permanent loss of hearing, a condition known as acoustic trauma[24]. High noise levels have also been shown to be associated with an increased risk of injuries at work[25].

EXAMPLES

◆ In Thailand, weavers exposed to 100dBA had more hearing loss than other textile workers[26]. Forty per cent. never used ear protection. In a plastic bag factory 80% of workers exposed to 98dBA never used ear protection, mainly because none was provided[27]. There was a significant relationship between the high noise level and hearing loss at 4 KHz.

◆ The number of persons with noise-induced hearing loss is the highest of the reported occupational diseases in Singapore. A survey of small factories revealed that 38% of workers were exposed to noise above 85dBA in the work place. The figure for Hong Kong was 42%, Korea 83% and the Philippines 92%[28].

Many occupational hazards, including hearing loss, are compounded by exposure to various industrial chemicals such as heavy metals and organic solvents. When two or more hazards are present, their combined effect should be given primary consideration[29].

> **EXAMPLE**
>
> ◆ The combination of chemicals, noise and heat is a particularly serious hazard of the electroplating and semiconductor industries[29].

Heat is an additional source of hazard. High temperatures impose a thermal load on workers, reducing productivity and increasing injuries. Industrial processes using heat also create a fire hazard and can cause the explosion of gases and dusts in the confined spaces of factories.

Exposure to heavy metals occurs in many industrial processes including welding, smelting, engraving, lithography and photography[30]. Women are especially at risk[31]. Chronic exposure to low concentrations increases the incidence of stillbirth, interrupted pregnancies and other complications of pregnancy including foetal damage[32].

> **EXAMPLE**
>
> ◆ The incidence of miscarriage in Europe is higher among women working in the chemical sector[33].

The semi-conductor industry uses extremely hazardous chemicals and processes[34]. The basic production steps are crystal doping, integrated circuit fabrication and packaging. The chemicals used in crystal doping include antimony, arsenic, chromium and phosphine. The associated health hazards include skin irritation, respiratory disease and various cancers. The chemicals used in integrated circuit fabrication include corrosive acids and strong solvents. The associated health hazards include corrosive ulceration, narcosis, mutagenicity, teratogenicity and damage to internal organs. Packaging chemicals include epoxy resins that can cause severe dermatitis and allergic reactions. Many of the gases used in these processes are also flammable or explosive and must be stored in high pressure cylinders. Some of the liquids react violently with water.

Electric arc welders are exposed to damaging levels of ultraviolet radiation[35,36]. Traumatic eye injuries are common in the metal-working industries[37], especially grinding and welding. Simple methods of eye protection are available but frequently are not used[35].

EXAMPLES

◆ A study of welders in the USA determined that a doubling of exposure to UV-B radiation led to a 60% increase in the risk of cortical cataract[38].

◆ A European study noted that 64% of workers with eye injuries had not been using any form of eye protection, even where it was mandatory. 20% had sustained two or more eye injuries within twelve months[39]. A UK study noted that 70% of patients attending an eye clinic had sustained the injury at work, 1.8% required hospitalization[40].

Although personal protective equipment is available, it should not be seen as the first line of prevention. It is usually uncomfortable, hinders movement or vision and may not be maintained in a proper condition. Environmental controls are generally more effective than personal protection equipment. These include extractor fans to remove dust, ventilation to improve airflow, enclosure to prevent exposure to dangerous machines, substitution to prevent exposure to toxic substances and safety switches to prevent machinery being switched on while limbs are at risk.

Income generating projects for the poor are often a component of development assistance. These are expected to have a beneficial health impact through increased income. However, the associated occupational health hazards should be considered.

Many people working at home or in small informal enterprises use chemicals that should only be used under carefully controlled conditions with special safety equipment[4].

Serious health hazards abound in small factories employing primarily women and among women doing piecework at home[1]. Women working in factories are less likely to breast-feed their children, contributing to infant diarrhoea. Women are often employed in export industries such as electronics that require accurate repetitive tasks. The enforcement of occupational health standards is often particularly lax in export industry, resulting in acute poisoning, chronic conjunctivitis, eye-strain, migraine, arthritis, lung disease and fatigue. These hazards are offset by higher incomes that may reduce the prevalence of poverty-related diseases. The risks of congenital abnormalities associated with handling toxic chemicals remain largely undocumented.

> **EXAMPLE**
>
> ◆ A survey of workers from small industries in Korea in 1975 concluded that: 42% of workers from lead smelter and accumulator factories had signs of lead poisoning; 10% of workers using solvents had suspected intoxication; 18% of all workers had symptoms of occupational diseases. Tuberculosis prevalence was up to 26% in pneumoconiotics, compared to 3% in the total working population[19]. Frequency rates began to fall in 1981 after new laws were introduced.
>
> In 1987, 71% of reported occupational disease was coal miner's lung disease, 28% was noise induced disease, the remainder was due to lead, solvent, chromium, mercury and other chemical poisoning. Noise levels were highest in the shipbuilding, automobile, steel and mining industries. The case detection rate was about half that of Japan. Air samples of asbestos fibre concentrations in associated manufacturing industry were well above acceptable thresholds[41].

Many countries do not possess the staff or technology required to monitor levels of contamination in the air, water or workforce.

Metal ores and their natural contaminants, such as arsenic and lead, frequently receive primary processing and smelting in the country of origin. Problems of acute arsenic poisoning and long-term carcinogenic risk should be addressed.

3.2 MENTAL DISORDER

The relationship between psychosocial factors at work and impaired mental well-being has been demonstrated repeatedly in many countries[42].

Mass production work is characteristically monotonous and under stimulating[43]. The consequences include ill health, absenteeism, mass hysteria, alienation and occupational injuries [42,44,45,46,47,48].

Studies in Egypt have demonstrated considerable substance abuse by industrial workers[49]. Abuse was more common among skilled than unskilled workers[50]. Workers explained that they abused drugs in order to work longer hours[51]. Prevalence was highest among drivers and construction workers[52]. This has implications for increased traumatic injury.

The physical design of the work place can result in social deprivation by decreasing group cohesion and support. The opposite extreme may be equally stressful, namely when the situation is characterised by total lack of privacy[53]. Psychosocial distress is also associated with a worker's fear of exposure to life threatening chemical hazards and other dangers[54].

4   AGRICULTURAL PROCESSING INDUSTRIES

In adition to the general range of occupational hazards of industry, including injury and noise, some specific health hazards of agricultural processing industries require description. These hazards are associated with non-communicable disease.

4.1   NON-COMMUNICABLE DISEASE

Industrial development is often associated with the agricultural sector where commodities such as tea, coffee, sugar, jute and pyrethrum are processed. Such processing plants expose labour to silica dust, a variety of allergens and spore contaminants that can cause or aggravate lung disease[55,56,57]. Women form a high and poorly paid proportion of such labour. There is evidence that the prevalence of chronic respiratory symptoms is higher in women workers, although they are usually non-smokers[58]. Exposure to tobacco dust causes respiratory, skin, eye and gynaecological problems[59]. Protective clothing is often not provided.

EXAMPLES

◆ Workers exposed to grain dust in South Africa had a high prevalence of irreversible loss of lung function compared with controls. There was a high prevalence of cough, expectoration, wheeze and watery eyes in grain workers. These symptoms were not related to duration of employment or smoking habits[57].

◆ Rice millers in Malaysia suffer from acute and chronic irritation of the eyes, skin and upper respiratory tract; allergic responses such as nasal catarrh and asthma; and lung changes associated with dust induced lung disease[60].

A respiratory disease is associated with handling of bagasse. Bagasse is the residual fibre of sugar cane after the juice has been extracted. It is usually compressed and stored for drying. It is used for board and paper making. Fungi and bacteria grow in the bagasse and cause an allergic reaction. It is estimated that the disease develops in up to 50% of those exposed. It can be prevented by modified storage of bagasse[61].

Large quantities of water are used and organic contaminants may be discharged into surface waters that are used for domestic supply. Post-harvest processing of agricultural produce can cause more severe river pollution than discharge of raw sewage[62]. The effect of discharges on downstream communities and on fish is seasonal. Much produce is processed during the dry season when temperatures are highest and river flow rates are lowest[63].

TABLE I   Examples of occupational hazards associated with agricultural processing

Produce	Exposure	Health Risk
Beedi cigarettes, India	Tobacco and bad posture	Poisoning and postural problems
Coir, India	Heavy dust	Dermatitis, hyperkeratosis, respiratory disease
Cashew nuts, Kerala	Fumes and corrosive liquids	Dermatitis, abscesses, boils, respiratory disease
Rice	Dust	Acute and chronic irritation of eyes, nose, lungs and skin
Pineapples, Swaziland	Acidic fruit juices	Dermatitis
Bagasse	Fibre	Respiratory disease
Textiles	Dust	Respiratory disease

Textile processing produces large quantities of air-borne fibres that cause chronic lung disease, such as byssinosis in cotton workers. This can reactivate latent tuberculosis.

EXAMPLES

◆ Many of the Colombian population derive drinking water directly from rivers. Rivers were highly polluted by discharges from the coffee, sugar and paper industry. A system of fining was introduced that has encouraged producers to recycle some of the waste[62].

◆ In the cotton industry in Sudan, byssinosis prevalence is as high as 49%[64]. Other respiratory symptoms are common, but no increase in tuberculosis was reported[65]. Byssinosis prevalence was much higher in Manchester cotton mills than in artificial fibre mills[66].

◆ Kapok workers in Sri Lanka are reported to develop chronic bronchitis and mill fever. Paprika splitters and chili millers are also known to develop allergic respiratory disease[67].

◆ Raw silk processors are exposed to a dust derived from the gum which binds silk strands together. In Sri Lanka occupational asthma was associated with degree of exposure to this dust[68].

◆ In China, pneumoconiosis was reported in silk workers[69].

5   STORED PRODUCE

The international trade in food products depends on an increasingly complex technology. Many countries lack the necessary regulations and enforcement to ensure product integrity. Refrigerated products are especially important[4].

5.1   COMMUNICABLE DISEASE

Stored food products are susceptible to contamination by mycotoxins, such as aflatoxin. These are produced by fungi at specific conditions of temperature and humidity[70]. Storage of produce in plastic bags is especially dangerous. The many adverse effects can include reduced effectiveness of immunization programmes and increased susceptibility to communicable diseases such as measles and HIV. Animal experiments provide evidence of interactions between malaria and aflatoxins[71,72].

Listeriosis, caused by the bacteria *Listeria monocytogenes*, is of great concern to the food industry. The bacteria can be found in a variety of dairy products, leafy vegetables, fish and meat products. It can grow in refrigerated foods and is heat resistant. Those predisposed to listeriosis include the immuno-compromised, pregnant women and their foetuses. Meningitis, spontaneous abortion and septicaemia are the primary manifestations of the disease[73]. The introduction of a refrigerated food industry could result in an increase in the incidence of listeriosis.

EXAMPLE

◆ A recent outbreak of listeriosis in California was linked to the consumption of Mexican-style soft cheese and involved more than 300 cases, 30% of which were fatal[73].

5.2   NON-COMMUNICABLE DISEASE

The adverse effects of contamination by mycotoxins, such as aflatoxin, can include acute fatal poisoning, immunosuppression and long term risks of liver cancer[74]. The toxin is an extremely stable molecule that is unaffected by cooking, fermenting or pickling. There is no reliable method of decontamination. The fungi can infect growing crops as a consequence of pest damage and produce toxins before, during or after harvest. Outbreaks of aflatoxicosis are common in farm animals and the toxins can carry over to meat and milk. Aflatoxins cross the placenta and are excreted in mother's milk[75]. Powdered milks may also contain aflatoxins. Occupational exposure occurs in workers of stored products.

EXAMPLE

◆ An outbreak of acute fatal liver disease in India was associated with ingestion of heavily aflatoxin-contaminated maize. Geographical variation in liver cancer prevalence has been associated with daily aflatoxin intake[74].

The export of stored food products by developing countries to industrialized countries is jeopardised by mycotoxins. Products are tested on arrival and may be condemned. Turkish fig exports to the EC were affected in 1989. There are reports of condemned foodstuffs being resold to poorer countries. Emergency food relief supplies can also become contaminated while awaiting trans-shipment.

5.3 MALNUTRITION

Aflatoxin exposure is suspected to be a common cause of kwashiorkor, in association with protein-energy malnutrition[76].

6 LEATHER TANNING AND FINISHING

About 250 chemicals are used in tanneries including tannin, chromium and alum as well as other acids, alkalis, solvents, oils, finishes and dyes.

Materials that can appear in tannery wastes include: hair, hide scraps, pieces of flesh, blood, manure, dirt, salts, lime, soluble proteins, sulphides, amines, chromium salts, tannin, soda ash, sugars and starches, oils, fats, greases, surface agents, mineral acids, dyes and solvents. Some of these are hazardous to health.

Particulate matters and hydrogen sulphide are the two potential gaseous discharges of significance[77]. Air pollution is mainly caused by the discharge of chemicals associated with unhairing liquid and pickling operations.

EXAMPLE

◆ A study monitoring air pollution in the residential area of Chiampo Valley in northern Italy, where about 150 tanneries are located, found that the highest concentration of hydrogen sulphide was detected within 1 kilometre downwind of 40 tanneries[78].

Measures for control and treatment of wastes are available. Shavings produced when processing hides into leather can be treated to extract the chromium contents for recycling. This leaves a waste by-product which can be used as glue, animal food or fertilizer for non-edible crops. However most of these measures and regulations regarding the disposal of waste are ignored, and most wastes are just dumped in the environment especially in developing countries[79].

6.1   COMMUNICABLE DISEASE

The main communicable health hazard of the leather industry is anthrax.

6.2   NON-COMMUNICABLE DISEASE

The main non-communicable health hazard of the leather industry is dermatitis from contacts with chemicals and hides.

Chromium can cause indolent and painful chrome ulcers of the skin and nasal septum in addition to dermatitis.

Other significant hazards associated with the leather industry include exposure to excessive dust, toxic chemicals, noise and reproductive hazards[33].

EXAMPLES

◆ In Jajmau, an industrial slum of Kanpur in India, occupational morbidity was 28% among tannery workers[80].

◆ A study of 252,147 live birth babies delivered in Scotland between 1981–1984 found that women who worked in leather had rates of pre-term delivery and low birth weight which were 50% higher than in most other female manual workers[81].

◆ In Montreal, Canada, a survey of pregnancy in leather workers found a significant excess of stillbirths[82].

Dust, produced in many leather working processes may be responsible for causing chronic bronchitis[83]. Asthma causing agents used in tanning include casein, chromium salts, paraphenylendiamine and formaldehyde[84].

Hydrogen sulphide gas is released through mixing of sulphides and chromic acid. Though such contact is avoidable, fatal incidents have occurred[83].

A number of substances used in the leather industry, such as azo dyes and chromium, are genotoxic leading to mutagenic and carcinogenic effects[33,79,85,86]. Exposure to atmospheric chromate may cause bronchogenic carcinoma with a latent period of 10–15 years[79].

> **EXAMPLE**
>
> ◆ Excess level of bladder, nasal, laryngeal and lung cancer and leukaemia have been reported in leather workers in several countries[87,88,89].

6.3 INJURY

The major injuries are caused by machinery, falls on slippery floors, and chemical burns from acid, alkalis and chromic acid.

> **EXAMPLE**
>
> ◆ Both injury and illness rates are considerably higher in the tannery industry than the average for all other industries. In the USA, in 1975, leather tanning and finishing workers had an incidence rate of 20.9 total injuries per 100 full time workers against an incidence rate of 12.5 total injuries in this category for all manufacturing workers (time unit not cited). In the category of occupational illnesses, the incidence rate per 100 full time workers was 2.4 for leather tanning and finishing workers, against an incidence rate of 0.5 for all manufacturing workers[83].

7 TOBACCO

7.1 GENERAL

See also Agricultural Processing Industries, section 3 and Agriculture, chapter 6, Choice of Crop.

In the developing world the health consequences of smoking may be exacerbated by synergism with endemic infectious diseases and other environmental hazards. This may lead to an increase in certain cancers. Reported linkages include tuberculosis and lung carcinoma, schistosomiasis and bladder carcinoma and occupational exposure to organic dusts, uranium or asbestos and cancer[90].

7.2 NON-COMMUNICABLE DISEASE

There has been an increase in trade in tobacco in recent years as countries have developed and entered economic trade on a global scale. From 1960 to 1980 cigarette consumption rose by 400% in India and by 300% in Papua New Guinea. Exports from the West, particularly the United States, to developing countries are high[90]. A number of studies in Europe have shown that workers exposed to tobacco dust are at increased risk of a variety of respiratory symptoms such as wheeze and dyspnoea.

EXAMPLES

◆ In Pakistan, where tobacco is now the most important cash crop, cigarette consumption has been growing at 8% annually[91]. Lung cancer is now the most commonly reported fatal cancer whereas oral, metastatic and skin cancers were most common ten years ago[90]. A leading aid agency recently gave a $60 million loan to Pakistan for growing tobacco[91].

◆ In Bangladesh, perinatal mortality is 270 per 10,000 for children of smoking mothers, more than twice the rate for children of non-smoking mothers[90].

---

8   TOURISM

8.1   COMMUNICABLE DISEASE

Tourism is a major source of hard currency for many countries. It creates a contact point between two diverse groups of vulnerable people: the tourist and the local community. The health of tourists is at risk due to their own behaviour (eg: sexual promiscuity[92], consumption of unhygienically pre-pared foods) and endemic health hazards (eg: diarrhoea and chloroquine resistant malaria).

The health education of tourists is frequently inadequate. A recent review[93] noted that only two thirds of travel brochures refer to health hazards. Only 16% of British passengers are advised of malaria risks by their travel agent; less than 50% attending a pre-travel health clinic were aware of malaria transmission; about 50% of tourists used malaria chemoprophylaxis effec-tively. Less than 50% of passengers in a survey were aware of the high HIV prevalence in the country of their destination.

Regional authorities recognise that endemic health hazards may threaten the entire tourist industry. For this reason they may seek to deny that those hazards exist.

Travellers' diarrhoea affects 30–50% of international travellers to developing countries of whom 30% may be confined to bed. Drug prophylaxis is associated with a number of adverse reactions and dietary avoidance is frequently ineffective[93].

Malaria prophylaxis for the tourist depends on well known drugs such as chloroquine, malaprim and paludrine (proguanil). Unfortunately, drug re-sistance is spreading rapidly throughout the world so that the recommended

EXAMPLES

◆ Annual visitors to Haiti dropped from 70,000 to 10,000 when AIDS was recognised[92].

◆ Thailand earns over $1 billion p.a. from tourism, spends $170 million on tourist promotion, and has a thriving sex industry. By 1987 some 3% of male sex workers were HIV positive. More recently there has been a rapid increase[92].

◆ A survey in Sri Lanka indicated that 10% of tourists had local sexual contact[92].

◆ It has been estimated that up to 100,000 women are employed in the 'hospitality industry' in Manila. The Philippines are trying to expand tourism and face the same problem as Thailand in the control of HIV. The inter-regional movements of sex-orientated tourists, primarily from the more affluent countries, highlight the potential for the international transmission of HIV[94].

prophylactic regime becomes ineffective. One response is to change to newer drugs such as mefloquine. However, in South East Asia almost all available drugs are now ineffective. In a survey of general practitioners less than 14% were fully aware of the distribution of chloroquine resistant malaria[93].

The development of centrally air-conditioned hotels and office buildings contributes to an increase in Legionnaire's disease, a serious form of pneumonia. The micro-organism grows in the water cooling towers and is distributed in water droplets.

The local community is at risk of acquiring exotic infections from tourists (eg: HIV infection).

8.2 MALNUTRITION

Disruption of the local environment and economy threatens food security. Tourism introduces a demand for basic foods that raises the price in local markets and makes those foods unavailable to local consumers. Development of coastal wetlands for tourism changes the flow of nutrients and reduces the fish stocks on which local fishing communities depend. On the other hand, the local community benefits from new roads and the opportunity of employment.

8.3 MENTAL DISORDER

Tourism can undermine the culture of remote communities, introducing the diseases of affluence and psycho-social disorder.

EXAMPLE

◆ In Micronesia many young adult males 'drink to get drunk'. The availability of alcohol is encouraged and there is increasing promotion by importers and distributers aimed at the young and at women. Tourism is cited as one risk factor and traffic crashes and collisions as one consequence [95].

---

9 REFERENCES

1 D E C Cooper Weil, A P Alicbusan, J F Wilson, M R Reich, and D J Bradley, "The Impact of Development Policies on Health: A Review of the Literature." (World Health Organization, Geneva 1990).

2 World Health Organization Commission on Health and Environment, "Report of the Panel on Industry." (World Health Organization, Geneva 1992).

3 V T Covello, and R S Frey, "Technology-based environmental health risks in developing nations." *Tech Forecast Soc Change*. 1990, 37:159–179.

4 World Health Organization Commission on Health and Environment, "Our Planet, Our Health." (World Health Organization, Geneva 1992).

5 J LaDou, "The export of industrial hazards to developing countries." in-*Occupational Health in Developing Countries, Ed. J Jeyaratnam.* (Oxford University Press, Oxford 1992).

6 D Weir, "The Bhopal Syndrome: Pesticides, Environment and Health." (Earthscan Publications, London 1988).

7 H R Sobral, "Air pollution and respiratory diseases in children in Sao Paulo, Brazil." *Soc Sci Med*. 1989, 29:8:959–964.

8 J D Spengler, J Ware, M Schwab, H Ozkaynak, J Samet, and G Wagner, "Kanawha county health study." *Am Rev of Resp Dis Part 2*. 1990, 14:4:A77.

9 C A Pope, "Respiratory disease associated with community air pollution and a steel mill, Utah valley." *Am J Public Health*. 1989, 79:5:623–628.

10 Third World Network, "Toxic Terror." (Third World Network, Penang, Malaysia 1989).

11 R W Findley, "Pollution control in Brazil." *Ecol Law Qtrly*. 1988, 15:1:1–68.

12 J C P Pimenta, "Multinational corporations and industrial pollution in Sao Paulo, Brazil." in-*Multinational Corporations, Environment and the Third World, Ed. C S Pearson.* (Duke University Press, Durham 1987).

13 V Thomas, "Pollution Control in Sao Paulo, Brazil: Costs, Benefits and Effects on Industrial Location." (November 1981) The World Bank. Staff Working Paper No.501.

14 S W Cai, "Cadmium exposure and health effects among residents in an irrigation area with ore processing wastewater." *Sci Total Environ*. 1990, 90:67–73.

15 T Suzuki, and R Ohtsuka, "Proceedings of the International Symposium on Health Impact of Rapid Industrialization and Urbanization in Asia and the Pacific and its Public Health Activities." *J Human Ergol*. 1990, 19

16 V Gennaro, M S Tocherman, F Merlo, M Donithan, and M Constatini, "Effect of specific shipyard occupations on lung function." *Am Rev of Resp Dis Part 2*. 1990, 141:4:A595.

17 W D O Sakari, and A S Mubisi, "Work conditions and effect of lead on the health of workers." *East Afr Med J.* 1983, 60:8:565–571.

18 D Muangman, "Public health activities and health impact of rapid industrialization and urbanization in Thailand." *J Human Ergol.* 1990, 19:213–218.

19 M A El-Batawi, "Special problems of occupational health in the developing countries." in-*Occupational Health Practice*, Ed. R S F Schilling. 2nd ed., (Butterworths, London 1981).

20 A Zwi, Personal communication.

21 L I M Dharmawardene, "Finger clubbing in match factory workers in Fiji." *Ceylon Med J.* 1991, 36:73–76.

22 K H Phua, "Health and socio-economic development in Singapore: impact of rapid industrialization and occupational health activities." *J Human Ergol.* 1990, 19:145–161.

23 OHSC, "The prevalence of pneumoconiosis in four industrial establishments: a pilot study." (1990) First National Occupational Safety and Health Congress. Philippines. Occupational Health and Safety Centre.

24 I J Mackenzie, and A W Smith, Personal communication.

25 P A Wilkins, and W I Acton, "Noise and accidents – a review." *Ann Occup Hyg.* 1982, 25:3:249–260.

26 P Chavalitsakulchai, T Kawakami, U Kongmuang, P Vivatjestsadawut, and W Leongsrisook, "Noise exposure and permanent hearing loss of textile workers in Thailand." *Ind Health.* 1989, 27:4:165–173.

27 P Chavalitsakulchai, and H Shahnavaz, "The need for a participatory conservation programme for the reduction of noise exposure to Thai female workers." *Asia Pac J Public Hlth.* 1989, 3:310–314.

28 S C Foo, K C Lun, and L C Tan, "The Environmental aand Health Conditions in selected small-scale industrial sites in Asia: Regional Report." (1985) IDRC, Canada.

29 World Health Organization, "Combined Exposures to Chemicals." (1983) World Health Organization. Health Aspects of Chemical Safety: Interim Document No. 11.

30 B Nemery, "Metal toxicity and the respiratory tract." *Eur Respir J.* 1990, 3:2:202–219.

31 W N Rom, "Effects of lead on the female and reproduction: a review." *Mount Sinai J Med.* 1976, 43:5:542–552.

32 K Hemminki, P Kyyronen, M Niemi, K Koskinen, M Sallmen, and H Vainio, "Spontaneous abortions in an industrialized community in Finland." *Am J Public Health.* 1983, 73:1:32–37.

33 G Marinova, "Problems of interrupted pregnancy among working women." *Akush Ginekol Sofia.* 1978, 17:6:412–417.

34 C S Chelton, M Glowataz, and J A Mosovsky, "Chemical hazards in the semi-condutor industry." *IEEE transactions on Education.* 1991, 34:3:269–288.

35 C Hanke, and H Karsten, "Cataract in welders: contribution of occupational exposure, references for recognition as an occupational disease and presentation of preventive measures." *Z Gesamte Hyg.* 1990, 36:2:110–113.

36 B L Diffey, "Human exposure to ultraviolet radiation." *Semin Dermatol.* 1990, 9:2–10.

37 M R Reesal, R M Dufresne, D Suggett, and B C Alleyne, "Welder eye

injuries." *J Occup Med.* 1989, 31:12:1003–1006.

38 H R Taylor, "Ultraviolet radiation and the eye: an epidemiologic study." *Trans Am Ophthalmol Soc.* 1990, 87:802–253.

39 V T Bakholdt, and D Illum, "Occupational eye injuries." *Ugeskr Laeger.* 1990, 152:13:917–919.

40 C J Macewen, "Eye injuries: a prospective survey of 5671 cases." *Brit J Ophthalmol.* 1989, 73:11:888–894.

41 N W Paik, "Industrial hygiene in Korea." *J Human Ergol.* 1990, 19:129–144.

42 International Labour Office, "Psychosocial Factors at Work: Recognition and Control." *Occupational Safety and Health Series, vol. 56,* (International Labour Office, Geneva 1986).

43 J F O'Hanlon, "Boredom: Practical consequences and a theory." *Acta Psychologica.* 1981, 49:53–82.

44 P K Chew, W H Phoon, and H A Mae-Lim, "Epidemic hysteria among some factory workers in Singapore." *Singapore Med J.* 1976, 17:10–15.

45 C R Walker, and R H Guest, "The Man On The Assembly Line." (Harvard University Press, 1952).

46 R Blauner, "Alienation and Freedom: The Factory Worker and His Industry." (University of Chicago Press, Chicago 1964).

47 A G Zdravomyslov, and V A Yadov, "Effects of vocational distinctions on attitude to work." in-*Industry and Labour in the USSR,* Ed. GV Osipov. (Tavistock Pub., London 1966).

48 H L Wilensky, "Family life cycle, work and the quality of life: Reflections on the roots of happiness, despair and indifference in modern society." in-*Working Life: A Social Science Contribution to Work Reform,* Ed. B Gardell and G Johansson. (Wiley, London 1981).

49 S M Wassif, M H Fawzy, A H Abdel Karim, A R Abo El-Seoud, A R Ahmed-Refat, M S El Sadawi, and M M Nassif, "Some epidemiological features of addiction among industrial workers in Zagazig Area, Sharkia Governorate." *Egyptian Journal of Occupational Medicine.* 1990, 14:1:13–24.

50 I M Soueif, F A Yunis, and M S Taha, "Extent and patterns of drug abuse and its associated factors in Egypt." *Bull Narcotics.* 1988, 38:1:113–120.

51 F H Zaki, M A Ghoneim, and I M Yehyia, "The problem of drug abuse; impact on medical, psychological and sociocultural aspects in Egypt." *Mansourah Medical Bulletin.* 1984, 12:2:35–44.

52 S El-Bestar, "Extent and pattern of drug dependence in some occupations." *Egyptian Journal of Occupational Medicine.* 1990, 14:1:127–137.

53 L Levi, "Stress in Industry: Causes, Effects and Prevention." *Occupational Safety and Health Series, vol. 51,* (International Labour Office, Geneva 1984).

54 L Levi, "Preventing Work Stress." (Addison-Wesley, Reading 1981).

55 P Blanc, "Environmental health and development in a developing country: Rwanda, a case study." *J Publ Hlth Policy.* 1984, 6:271–288.

56 T T Ye, D M Lewis, W G Sorenson, and S A Olenchock, "Inflammatory potential of grain dust." *Biomed Environ Sci.* 1988, 1:1:115–124.

57 D Yach, J Myers, D Bradshaw, and S R Benatar, "A respiratory epidemiologic survey of grain mill workers in Cape Town, South Africa." *Am Rev of Resp Dis.* 1984, 131:505–510.

58 E Zuskin, F Valic, and Z Skuric, "Respiratory function in coffee workers." *Brit J Indust Med.* 1979, 36:117–122.

59 Nag Anjali, "Occupational Health Hazards for Women in India." (1986) National Institute of Occupational Health, Women's Cell, Ahmedabad, Gujerat, India.

60 H H Lim, Z Domala, S Joginder, S H Lee, C S Lim, and C M Abu Bakar, "Rice millers' syndrome: a preliminary report." *Brit J Ind Med.* 1984, 41:445–449.

61 H Phool Chund, "Health and safety in agriculture: the sugarcane industry." *African Newsletter on Occupational Health and Safety.* 1991, 1:3:83–85.

62 A Agarwal, J Kimondo, G Moreno, and J Tinker, "Water, Sanitation, Health – for All? Prospects for the International Drinking Water Supply and Sanitation Decade, 1981–1990." (Earthscan Publications, London 1981).

63 S Cairncross, and R G Feachem, "Environmental Health Engineering in the Tropics: An Introductory Text." (John Wiley & Sons, Chichester 1983).

64 M Khogali, "Industrial health problems in developing countries: types of risks and their prevention." *J Trop Med Hyg.* 1970, 73:272.

65 M A A El Karim, and A A El Hag, "Byssinosis and tuberculosis in the cotton industry in Sudan." *East Afr Med J.* 1985, 62:7:491–500.

66 D Fishwick, F Fletcher, C A Pickering, R Riven, and N Raza, "A cross-sectional study of respiratory symptoms in textile spinning mills." *Am Rev of Resp Dis Part 2.* 1990, 141:4:A248.

67 D K Sekimpi, "Occupational health services for agricultural workers." in-*Occupational Health in Developing Countries, Ed. J Jeyaratnam.* (Oxford University Press, Oxford 1992).

68 C G Uragoda, and P N B Wijekoon, "Asthma in silk workers." *J Soc Occup Med.* 1991, 41:140–142.

69 Liu Tie-min, "Tussah silk pneumoconiosis: investigation and experiment study." *Am Rev of Resp Dis Part 2.* 1990, 141:4:A248.

70 World Health Organization, "Mycotoxins." (1979) World Health Organization. Environmental Health Criteria No.11.

71 R G Hendrickse, S M Lamplugh, and B G Maegraith, "Influence of aflatoxin on nutrition and malaria in mice." *Trans R Soc Trop Med Hyg.* 1986, 80:5:846–7.

72 R H Young, R G Hendrickse, S M Maxwell, and B G Maegraith, "Influence of aflatoxin on malarial infection in mice." *Trans R Soc Trop Med Hyg.* 1988, 82:4:559–560.

73 J M Farber, and J Z Losos, "Listeria monocytogenes: a foodborne pathogen." *Can Med Assoc J.* 1988, 138:5:413–418.

74 R G Hendrickse, "Clinical implications of food contaminated by aflatoxins." *Ann Acad of Med (Singapore).* 1991, 20:1:84–90.

75 S M Maxwell, F Apeagyei, H R de Vries, D D Mwanmut, and R G Hendrickse, "Aflatoxins in breast milk, neonatal cord blood and sera of pregnant women." *J Toxicology – Toxin reviews.* 1989, 8:1&2:19–29.

76 R G Hendrickse, and S M Maxwell, "Aflatoxins and child health in the tropics." *J Toxicology – Toxin reviews.* 1989, 8:1&2:31–41.

77 The World Bank, "Environmental Guidelines." (The World Bank Environment Department, Washington 1988).

78 V Cocheo, "Environmental impact of tanning industry." *Med Lav.* 1990, 81:3:230–241.

79 K D G P Dodangoda, "Protein from toxic wastes." *ASEP Newsletter.* 1992, 8:1:6–7.

80 A Shukla, S Kumar, and F G Ory, "Occupational health and the environment in an urban slum in India." *Soc Sci Med*. 1991, 33:5:597–603.
81 S Sanjose, E Roma, and V Beral, "Low birthweight and preterm delivery, Scotland, 1981–84: effects of parents' occupation." *The Lancet*. 1991, 338:8764:428–431.
82 A D McDonald, and J C McDonald, "Outcome of pregnancy in leatherworkers." *Brit Med J (Clin Res Ed)*. 1986, 292:6526:979–982.
83 The World Bank, "Occupational Health and Safety Guidelines." (The World Bank Environment Department, Washington 1988).
84 J M Olaguibel, D Hernandez, P Morales, A Peris, and A Basomba, "Occupational asthma caused by inhalation of casein." *Allergy*. 1990, 45:4:306–308.
85 E Clonfero, P Venier, M Granella, and A G Levis, "Leather azo dyes: mutagenic and carcinogenic risks." *Med Lav*. 1990, 81:3:222–229.
86 E Clonfero, P Venier, M Granella, and A G Levis, "Identification of genotoxic compounds used in leather processing industry." *Med Lav*. 1990, 81:3:12–221.
87 W Ahrens, K H Jockel, W Patxak, and G Elsner, "Alcohol, smoking and occupational factors in cancer of the larynx: a case control study." *Am J Ind Med*. 1991, 20:4:477–493.
88 N Yamaguchi, S Watanabe, T Okubo, and K Takahashi, "Work-related bladder cancer risks in male Japanese workers: estimation of attributable fraction and geographical correlation analysis." *Jpn J Cancer Res*. 1991, 82:6:624–631.
89 A Seniori Costantini, E Merler, and R Saracci, "Epidemiologic studies on carcinogenic risk and occupational activities in tanning, leather and shoe industries." *Med Lav*. 1990, 81:3:184–211.
90 M Barry, "The influence of the US tobacco industry on the health, economy and environment of developing countries." *N Eng J Med*. 1991, 324:13:917–920.
91 K R Stebbins, "Transnational tobacco companies and health in underdeveloped countries: recommendations for avoiding a smoking epidemic." *Soc Sci Med*. 1990, 30:2:227–235.
92 The Panos Institute, "Aids and the Third World." (The Panos Institute, London 1988).
93 R H Behrens, "Protecting the health of the international traveller." *Trans R Soc Trop Med Hyg*. 1990, 84:5:611,612,629.
94 N Ford, and S Koetsawang, "The socio-cultural context of the transmission of HIV in Thailand." *Soc Sci Med*. 1991, 33:4:405–414.
95 World Health Organization, "Report on the Workshop on Alcohol and Drug Related Problems in Micronesia." (5–9 June, 1989) World Health Organisation. WHO/(WP)MNH/ICP/ADA/002.

chapter 13

1   INTRODUCTION

The following material is designed as a problem based learning exercise. It was originally developed for a training course jointly organised with the WHO/FAO/UNEP/UNCHS Panel on Environmental Management for Vector Control (PEEM) and the Danish Bilharziasis Laboratory (DBL). The course was entitled "Health Opportunities in Water Resource Development". The material was subsequently modified and tested in numerous courses at the Liverpool School of Tropical Medicine.

The objective is to provide a focused discussion for a multi-disciplinary audience, representing different public sectors, on the preparation of a rapid health impact assessment of a water resource development project.

1.1   CONTENTS

The chapter contains the following main components:

◆   A complete set of the handouts that are supplied to the participants, one at a time, during the exercise.

◆   A blank summary table that can be photocopied and completed.

◆   A tutor's note providing additional technical information.

1.2   PROCEDURE

The class is divided into small groups (maximum 6 per group) and ideally each group has a tutor. The role of the tutor is to facilitate while the group explores the scenario of a water resource development in the imaginary African Republic of San Serriffe. In each group, the participants debate a series of structured questions using the handouts for guidance. Time is allowed for private study in which members of the group research the answers to priority questions and then present the answers that they have discovered back to the group. Each group writes a final report.

1.3   TIMING

The exercise requires a whole day of discussion and private study plus several hours for report writing.

1.4 REFERENCE

The participants are provided with copies of this book. Additional technical information can be found in:

Birley, M H (1991). *Guidelines for forecasting the vector-borne disease implications of water resource development*. WHO/PEEM Series 2. WHO/CWS/91.3.
The Guidelines are available from WHO, and may also be obtained from the author in a hypertext format compatible with MS DOS Windows.

HANDOUT NUMBER 1:   Scenario

An Assessment of the Health Impact of Water Resource Development in San Serriffe

The imaginary Republic of San Serriffe has a woodland savanna environment. There are high mountains in the north and sea around the southern peninsula. The capital is called Villa Pica. The urban and rural communities are largely from different cultural backgrounds. The rural people are called Flong. They are subsistence agriculturalists who grow maize, keep pigs, goats and cows and gather other food from the woodlands.

The San Serriffe government want a development loan to build a hydropower and irrigation project. The ideal valley sites for the reservoir and fields have been identified in the southern foothills of the mountain range. About 12,000 Flong will have to be resettled.

A smaller hydropower scheme was completed ten years ago. The Flong community, 2,000 people from 20 villages, were displaced and resettled. Some were resettled as the workforce on a commercial irrigated wheat farm, in place of their subsistence agriculture.

Your Task

As part of the Environmental Impact Assessment, the donor agency wants you to assess the health impacts of the proposed project and to suggest health safeguards and mitigation measures. Please give priority to vector-borne diseases.

HANDOUT NUMBER 2:   How this Problem Based Exercise Will Be Organised

1   There will be no lecture. The tutor will facilitate – not teach.

2   The exercise will be divided into a series of steps, summarised in the Objectives.

3   Each step is accompanied by a handout. **Do not look at** the handout until you are asked to do so.

4   You will be encouraged to ask questions within the context of each step.

5   Some questions will be listed on each handout. These will refer either to the handout you have been given or, if <u>underlined</u>, to a handout you have not yet seen.

5   You will be encouraged to share your knowledge and experience with the group.

6   Time will be provided for you to research answers to the questions.

Outputs

a   A list of questions.
b   A report answering some of the questions.

What You Must Do

Please contribute to the discussion.
Please keep a written list of any questions that seem important to you.

First questions

1   Do you understand how the exercise will be organised?
2   <u>Do you understand what is meant by Health Impact Assessment?</u>

HANDOUT NUMBER 3:   Definition of Health Impact Assessment

Assessment   Examination in order to decide.

Health impact   Change in the frequency of some health indicators among the vulnerable community which is reasonably attributable to the project.

Development projects are designed to confer benefits on the community, including improved standards of living and health. There are sometimes unintended and indirect dis-benefits. These may affect the environment, the socio-economic condition or the health status of some communities.

Increases in ill-health represent a hidden cost of the project which must be borne by the health sector.

Health impact assessment (HIA) provides an early warning so that decision-makers can review and modify project plans and operations by negotiation.

Questions

1   Do you understand the definition?
2   What relevant information is there on the Handout describing the scenario?

HANDOUT NUMBER 4:   Objectives

By the end of the exercise you will be able to describe a procedure for assessing the health impact of a development project in the tropics. You will also be able to discuss some facts about health impacts.

The main sub-tasks are:
1   Agreeing a procedure
2   Identifying health hazards
3   Assessing the health risks associated with the health hazards
4   Deciding whether mitigation would be difficult
5   Presenting the results

Questions

What procedure should we use to assess health impact? Hint: this is a management problem.

HANDOUT NUMBER 5: A Health Impact Assessment Procedure

1. Decision by non-health specialist that a health impact assessment is needed.
2. A rapid assessment designed to spot important health risks and classify the project into one of three categories, as follows. *This is our task.*

Classification	Interpretation
A	Significant health impacts, mitigation difficult or requires full HIA or requires special budget
B	Significant health impacts, mitigation practical without special budget, may require HIA
C	No significant health impacts

3. A full health impact assessment, if necessary.

Questions

1. Why is the first decision made by a non-health specialist? *The answer is in Chapter 1.*
2. Why is step 2 needed before step 3? *The answer to this is also in Chapter 1.*
3. How would you define a health hazard and a health risk?

HANDOUT NUMBER 6:   Health Hazard and Risk

Health hazard   =   A potential for causing harm to people
Health risk   =   The likelihood that the potential is realised

Examples:

1   Malaria is a health hazard in the tropics. However, malaria is a very small health risk in the middle of many large cities in the tropics because of the absence of the mosquitoes which can transmit the infection.

2   Electrocution is a health hazard in your home. However, the risk of electrocution depends on:

- exposure of a person who is unaware of the hazard;
- a live wire;
- behaviour which causes simultaneous contact with the wire and with the earth.

Questions

1   What health hazards would you expect to be associated with development projects in general?

2   Can you group these into 4–5 main categories?

HANDOUT NUMBER 7:   Health Hazards of Development

Suggestion for one way of categorising health hazards associated with development.

Health hazard	Example of hazard or cause
Communicable disease	*Malaria, diarrhoea, respiratory infection*
Non-communicable disease	*Poisoning, pollution, dust*
Malnutrition	*Reduced subsistence foods*
Injury	*Traffic or occupational injury*
Mental disorder	*Substance abuse, stress*

Questions:

1   Do you have any health hazards that do not fit into these categories?
2   How could a development planner, with no health experience, decide whether a development project requires a health impact assessment?

HANDOUT NUMBER 8:   Project Screening

Screening tools are used by non-health specialists to identify projects
which may increase health risks. Once identified, these projects may
receive a partial, or full, health impact assessment. Projects are
identified on the basis of:

- Health sensitive locations
  *Identified from maps, local health records and knowledge of disease
  foci*
- Health sensitive components
  *Hazardous operations and materials; hazards previously associated
  with specific types of development.*

Questions

1   What kind of health hazards are commonly associated with water
     resource developments?
2   How could you find out if the project is in a health sensitive location?

HANDOUT NUMBER 9:   National Health Data, San Serriffe

Location:	**Sub-Saharan Africa**	
Accurate census 1975	Total population	663,224
	Villa Pica (the capital)	50,000
	Woj (town nearest project)	10,000
	Zapf (a town in district 4)	12,000

Area	10,000km^2
Highest mountain	6438m
Swamp in eastern coastal belt	
Mean day temperature	30°C

Special surveys have indicated the true disease prevalence rates[1] in lowland areas:

malaria prevalence rate	30% (97% *falciparum*)
schistosomiasis prevalence rate	20%

1986 case reports from the 4 districts, see attached maps, were as follows.

Districts of San Serriffe

Case reports 1986	1 excluding Villa Pica	2	3	4	Villa Pica
Malaria	19,000	13,000	10,000	1,000	2,000
Schistosomiasis	500	0	12,000	4,000	0
Filariasis	1,190	0	0	2,000	7,000
Sleeping sickness	0	20	0	0	0
Dengue	0	0	0	0	1,500
Population, approx.	317,477	50,000	245,747		50,000

Questions

1 Is there anything wrong with this data? Hint: consider under-reporting.
2 What should be the scope of the health impact assessment?

---

[1] Prevalence rate = existing cases at specified point of time / total population at risk
Incidence rate = new cases in specified period of time / total population at risk

Republic of San Serriffe - Africa   District boundaries

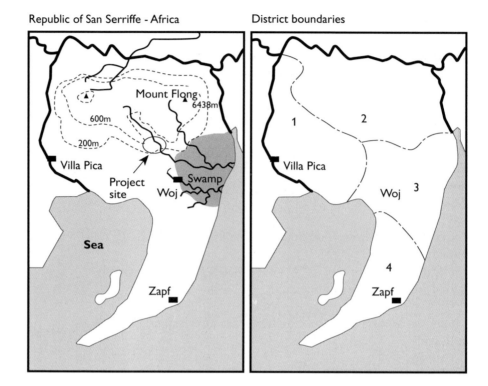

HANDOUT NUMBER 10:   Project Scoping

Scoping is the process of determining what to include and not include in the impact assessment. There are four main questions.

1   The health hazards to include

We shall restrict our assessment to vector-borne diseases.

2   The number of years into the future to include.

Some vector-borne diseases spread slowly through a community and may not become a widespread cause of ill-health for many years. Others spread very quickly and are an immediate cause of ill-health.

Example: Malaria is a "fast" disease but schistosomiasis is a "slow" disease.

3   The geographical boundaries to include

Vectors and infected hosts may move considerable distances.

Example: the vectors of river blindness can migrate 300km downwind. Mosquitoes fly about 2km between breeding and feeding sites. Migrant workers can come from different countries.

4   The people to consult

There will be a series of specialists and government officers who will be able to provide information. Is it also important to consult the affected community?

Questions

1   Define "vector-borne disease".
   Which vector-borne diseases should we include? Why?
2   What are the project stages and which ones should be included in the assessment?
3   Where would you draw the geographical boundaries?
4   After we have established the scope, how can we break the problem of making the assessment into its component parts?

HANDOUT NUMBER 11:   The three main components of the rapid assessment

1   Who is at risk of exposure to the health hazards
    (*the vulnerable communities*)?
2   Why are they at risk?
    (*What are the factors in the environment responsible for that
    exposure?*)
3   What are the health protection agencies capable of doing to safeguard
    health?

Questions

1   Can you supply an example of each of these three components?
2   List some of the communities who may be at risk in San Serriffe.

HANDOUT NUMBER 12:   Who is at risk?

Some, but not all, of the communities associated with the project in San Serriffe are listed.

Displaced: 12,000 Flong subsistence farmers including dependents will be displaced from the reservoir and irrigation sites. Many will be offered a resettlement site on the irrigation scheme, the rest will move onto the slopes of Mount Flong, or drift into town.

Settlers: 5,700 cash crop farmers plus dependents will be settled on the irrigation scheme. These will include some Flong and some town dwellers.

Fishing folk: 300 plus dependents will be attracted to the new reservoir from the coast.

Police: about 20 plus dependents – to regulate activities around the reservoir.

Electricity workers: 100 workers plus dependents to produce hydro-electricity and maintain the dam.

Irrigation management and agricultural extension: 10 workers plus dependents.

Existing health centre: 2 nurses and a technician plus dependents.

Existing school: 7 teachers, 4 assistants plus dependents.

Construction workers: 4,000 males for 2 years including 100 international.

Engineering consultants: international, 20 plus dependents.

Camp followers: 350 food sellers plus dependents; 40 professional sex workers plus dependents; 29 merchants plus dependents.

Seasonal labour for farmers: 3,700 plus dependents.

Others: loggers and poachers, an unknown number; churches – at least 2; tourists and tour operators; rich city people making holiday homes; land speculators; administrators; ordinary traders; surveyors.

Question

1   What is it about these communities that may expose them to vector-borne disease hazards?
2   What factors would you expect to find in the environment that we ought to consider? For example, what are the disease transmission pathways?

AN EXERCISE IN RAPID HEALTH IMPACT ASSESSMENT

HANDOUT NUMBER 13:   Why are they at risk?

Consider the environmental factors in San Serriffe associated with vector-borne disease transmission.

Seasonal rainfall averages 1000mm per annum. There are short and long rains with two annual malaria peaks.

The principal malaria vectors are:
Anopheles gambiae breeding in rainpools and other collections of temporary water;
Anopheles arabiensis which seems to favour irrigation schemes;
Anopheles funestus which breeds in more permanent water such as the swamps east of Woj. There is also a non-malaria vector that is extremely abundant and easily confused with the first two malaria vectors. Malaria is absent from altitudes above 600m.

The natural vegetation is a closed canopy savanna woodland. There are now extensive areas of grassland. Woodlands are surrounded by a mosaic of cultivated patches where domestic animals are sometimes kept, when tsetse flies are absent. There are plenty of **tsetse flies** in the woodland and in several districts wild game are abundant.
Snail vectors of **schistosomiasis** are particularly plentiful in the swamps east of the town of Woj.
Flong villages are permanent and usually sited in large clearings near streams. Houses are usually circular and constructed of mud and wattle. Pigs, cows and other small stock are kept close to the home. Maize is stored in outhouses. Domestic water is obtained from streams which are also used for washing and bathing.

Filariasis and **dengue** are largely restricted to the urban environment, at present.

Questions

1   What is it about project design and operation and peoples' behaviour in relation to the project, which exposes some community groups to vector-borne diseases?
2   What would you expect the health services and any other health protection agencies to be doing at present to protect health?

HANDOUT NUMBER 14:   What is being done to protect health?

The capabilities of the health service and other protection agencies in San Serriffe are limited. The following notes are NOT based on any real country.

The health service has been established for 100 years in San Serriffe. It maintains peripheral health centres and referral hospitals in Villa Pica. It supplies drugs such as chloroquine for malaria. Unfortunately, chloroquine resistance is widespread and chloroquine is often out of stock. There are some diagnostic laboratories but they are understaffed and short of equipment.

The health centres supply monthly statistical summaries to district headquarters. National health statistics (see Handout 9) are published annually but three years in arrears.

There is one malaria vector control unit based in Villa Pica. It travels to each district when its vehicles are functional.

There is one health education unit which provides family planning information.

There is no schistosomiasis control unit.

Trypanosomiasis control is run by the veterinary service. Most activity is directed to the important cattle ranches north of Mount Flong.

Dengue control units are under municipal control in the major towns.

Question

1   How could the capability of these services be strengthened?
2   Now that we have examined the three main components of health impact assessment, how should we combine them and present the results?

AN EXERCISE IN RAPID HEALTH IMPACT ASSESSMENT

HANDOUT NUMBER 15:   Summary Health Impact Assessment Table, An Example

Project Title	Wheat farm, commercial irrigation
Location	San Serriffe, Africa
Community group	Irrigation scheme farmers and labourers
Project stage of forecast	Early operation

Health hazard	Community vulnerability	Environmental factors	Health service capability	Health risk
Malaria *falciparum*	high	unchanged	good curative moderate preventative	high
Schistosomiasis	low	increasing	mainly curative some prevention	low but increase expected
Sleeping sickness	very low	very low	curative only	very low

JUSTIFICATION/EXPLANATION

Malaria hazard

Vulnerability: Widespread chloroquine resistance, widespread ignorance of causation, seasonally major cause of hospital admissions, project workforce partly recruited from town where there was more health care and less malaria, so they are very susceptible. Other part of workforce are local Flong who are a reservoir of infection.

Environment: *An. gambiae* is a small pool breeder. Overhead sprinkler irrigation being used with 600m arms – no surface pooling so no extra breeding sites.

Health service capability:
Curative: local clinics short of drugs and in poor repair, personnel salaries delayed. Good mission hospital 50km away had not been informed of labour influx.

HANDOUT NUMBER 15:   Summary Health Impact Assessment Table, An Example *(continued)*

Prevention: no residual house spraying; window screens being built on worker's housing; mosquito nets generally regarded as too expensive.

Surveillance: no routine, reliable data.

Summary health risk: Migrant workforce will experience initial increase in prevalence due to locality. Project will not increase mosquito vectors.

Schistosomiasis hazard (Bilharzia)

Vulnerability: Foci in streams and water holes where children love to bathe. Alternative bathing points were provided for the workforce.

Environment: Irrigation canal cement lined, smooth and steep sided which deters bathing. Extra care needed at drop structures (cement dams across irrigation canal with steps).

Health service capability:
Curative: local clinic had no drugs; mission hospital had supplies of a suitable drug.
Prevention: piped water supply to workers settlement.
Surveillance: no routine data.

Summary health risk: Human density increasing near potential foci. Cannot stop children bathing so expect increased prevalence.

Sleeping sickness hazard (Trypanosomiasis)

Vulnerability: Restricted to hunters going to remote areas. Not at project site.

Environment: Proximity of project site to Miombo woodland and game park. Tsetse fly population had declined because poachers had removed the game due to shortage of meat in nearby towns. Game was the reservoir host.

Health service capability:
Curative: mission hospital used to treating sporadic cases.
Prevention: none.
Surveillance: tsetse maps maintained for cattle development.

Summary health risk: No game, no reservoir, no transmission.

HANDOUT NUMBER 16:   Completing the health risk assessment table

Question

1 Can you fill in a similar summary table for the new hydropower project?
   A blank table pro-forma is available on the next page.
2 What justifications can you suggest for your conclusions?
3 On the basis of this rapid assessment, what else do we need to know in order to classify the project into one of the following three categories?

Classification	Interpretation
A	Significant health impacts, mitigation difficult or requires full HIA or requires special budget
B	Significant health impacts, mitigation practical without special budget, may require full HIA
C	No significant health impacts

4 In order to decide whether mitigation is difficult, what do we need to know about the opportunities for health risk management?

HANDOUT NUMBER 17:   Pro-forma

Summary Health Impact Assessment Table

Project title

Location

Community group

Project stage

Health hazards	Community vulnerability	Environ-mental factors	Capability of health service and other protection agencies	Health risks

HANDOUT NUMBER 18:   Opportunities for Health Risk Management

1   List some possible mitigation measures.

2   Group the mitigation measures as follows:

    a   Opportunities for modifying project design.
    b   Opportunities for modifying project operation and maintenance.
    b   Opportunities for incorporating environmental management measures.
    c   Opportunities for strengthening health services.

3   Categorise each measure as:

    a   Cheap or expensive.
    b   Easy or difficult.
    c   Socially acceptable or not acceptable.
    d   Maintenance cheap or expensive.

HANDOUT NUMBER 19:   Some mitigations in San Serriffe

Settlement location
Purpose is to reduce exposure to contaminated water and insect bites.
Design stage; cheap if government owns the land; socially acceptable if
distance to fields or other workplace is not excessive.

Piped water supply
Purpose is to reduce exposure to contaminated water.
Design stage; expensive but easy; socially acceptable.

Irrigation and drainage channel maintenance
Purpose is to improve water flow, prevent leakage and stagnation and
prevent vector breeding. Operation and maintenance stage, must be
repeated regularly.
Cheap if community participates. Difficult to motivate community.

Impregnated bednets
Purpose is to reduce exposure to insect bites. Construction or operation
stage. Relatively cheap, social acceptability varies. Low maintenance
cost.

Improved drug supplies
Purpose is to cure individuals who become clinically ill. Relatively
cheap until drug resistance develops. Can use volunteer health workers.
Difficult to maintain supplies.
Difficult to motivate health workers to provide consistent service
(especially laboratory diagnosis).

Irrigation and drainage channel design
Purpose is to prevent vector breeding.
Design stage. Expensive, requiring more structures made from concrete.
Socially acceptable.

Sanitation
Purpose is to ensure safe excreta disposal, prevent contamination of
open water and prevent filariasis vector breeding and fly breeding.
Construction stage. VIP latrines are relatively cheap(?). Require regular
maintenance. Social acceptability varies.

Pesticide spraying
Purpose is to kill vectors and reduce biting nuisance. Construction and
operation stages.
Relatively expensive, requires repetitive treatment. Social acceptability
varies.

Health education
Purpose is to inform the community about the scientific explanation of disease transmission so that they may be encouraged to modify their attitude and behaviour. Requires the training of trainers, their salaries and transport and repeated reiteration of the same message.

Questions

1   What constraints might apply to implementing the measures you have selected?

HANDOUT NUMBER 20: Constraints to Health Risk Management in San Serriffe

Environmental management

Design: The Chief Engineer is not enthusiastic about changing the designs of the irrigation scheme or reservoir which have taken six years to prepare. Careful negotiation would be required, well supported by facts.

Operation: The water tax collection system was designed to maximise the project's cost-benefit ratio. The tax will assist central government to pay back the loan. Any proposal to use water tax locally for project maintenance will require good justification.

Provision of health services

The Principal Medical Officer was interested to hear that a development project was planned. She immediately drew up a budget for the construction, staffing, operation and maintenance of 5 extra health centres. Negotiations are proposed to determine who will pay. The donor agency has expressed an interest but requires a clear justification.

Monitoring and surveillance

The donor agency has a requirement for project monitoring during the first five years of operation. This does not usually include the construction phase. The cost of additional monitoring must be minimised or the project may not yield a positive rate of return.

HANDOUT NUMBER 21: Report Presentation

Maximum length: 7 pages. Maximum time: 4 hours.
Divide up the task among the group.

Title
Names of writers
Date of assessment

1 Introduction (one paragraph)
   Who is the assessment for and what are they expected to do with it?

2 Summary Table listing all the hazards considered and the conclusions concerning risk (one page). *You may wish to repeat the table for each community group or for different project stages.* A blank table is available for you to use.

3 Explanation of the conclusions presented in the Summary Table. Under each disease discuss:
   a Communities at risk (one paragraph)
   b Environmental factors that change exposure (one paragraph)
   c Capabilities of the health service and other protection agencies (one paragraph)
   d Whether the health risk will increase, decrease or remain the same and how this conclusion was reached (one paragraph).

4 Analysis of the opportunities for health risk management (safeguards and mitigations). Distinguish between design and operation stages and consider whether each measure is cheap/expensive, easy/difficult, and socially acceptable/not acceptable). Headings include:
   a Opportunities for modifying the project design.
   b Opportunities for incorporating environmental management measures
   c Opportunities for strengthening health services (*what is inadequate and what can realistically be improved?*)

TUTOR'S NOTE

Summary Health Impact Assessment Table

Location	San Serriffe (Africa)
Project Type	Hydropower and irrigation
Date of assessment	September 1992
Project stage	

Health hazards	Community vulnerability	Environmental factors	Capability of health service and other agencies	Health risk associated with the project
Malaria *falciparum*	High in all communities	High transmission potential	Low	High and increasing
Schistosomiasis (*haematobium and mansoni*)	Especially important for children	High	Low	High and increasing
Sleeping sickness	High for poachers, loggers and gatherers	High transmission potential	Low	Low but increasing among secondary communities
Filariasis	Low	Low	Low	Low, but monitor at five yearly intervals
Dengue	Low	Low	Low	Low, monitor circulation between town and project

EXPLANATION/JUSTIFICATION

The objective of the exercise is to facilitate a discussion. The participants should use their imagination. Therefore, a model answer is deliberately not included. The following notes provide additional technical information. They do not refer to any real country but are based on observations made in various countries.

MALARIA

There is no animal reservoir. Chloroquine resistance is common.

Vulnerable community

All the communities are vulnerable to the risk of *falciparum* malaria. But not all the communities will experience a change in risk associated with the project. Some Flong communities have partial immunity, characterised by high childhood and low adult rates of clinical illness. Some migrant communities from Mount Flong, overseas workers from temperate regions, city traders and fishing folks are especially vulnerable due to absence of previous exposure. Knowledge of malaria transmission is mixed. Many Flong associate malaria with the spirit world. Primary school graduates accept the scientific explanation.

Construction phase: The construction workers, their dependents and camp followers will be exposed to the normal wet season malaria. Poor living conditions may increase their exposure to biting mosquitoes. The construction company will provide screened accommodation for its workforce.

Early operation phase: The vulnerability of farmers and labourers on the irrigation scheme will depend on the use made of nets and repellents, house design and location, residual house spraying, source reduction, night time activity and health education. High birth rates will produce a large group of vulnerable infants and children. Requirements of cash cropping may induce mothers to wean their babies earlier with subsequent loss of protective immunity.

Fishing communities around the margin of the reservoir: These are an informal community who must purchase their own protection. As they work at night they experience increased exposure to mosquito vectors. There is no health service provision for these informal settlers.

Displaced: Displaced communities who establish farms on the slopes of Mount Flong may have reduced access to health services. However, the altitudinal limit for malaria transmission is 600m on San Serriffe.

Government employees: Electricity workers and other government employees will be moving from an area of low risk to an area of increased risk.

Late operation phase: If malaria is not controlled partial immunity will probably develop following a period of high mortality. The birth rate will probably remain very high so there will always be large numbers of vulnerable children.

Environmental factors

The malaria vectors are normally widespread in rural areas during the wet season. During the dry season they may be restricted to the vicinity of permanent ponds, swamps and streams.

Breeding sites: There is no malaria vector breeding in the city of Villa Pica but breeding sites are found in agricultural areas of the peri-urban fringe. Current breeding sites are temporary rainpools, seepages and borrow pits. The alteration of surface waters associated with the project is expected to extend the wet season abundance by creating three new classes of breeding site.

Drawdown zone: The reservoir margins may not provide many breeding sites as a result of predation, wave action and steep banks. The mosquitoes will breed in vegetated, sheltered inlets. However, when water is extracted for power generation or irrigation the level may fluctuate unpredictably. On shallow shores drawdown will expose many km^2 of muddy pools. These will become breeding sites if they persist for more than 1–2 weeks.

Irrigation system: The rice fields themselves may only provide suitable breeding sites during the early transplantation phase. The shaded conditions and water quality associated with canopy closure may deter vector species. Seepages and weed choked irrigation/drainage ditches are important.

Roadside pools: Interruption of surface flow by road construction and formation of borrow pits will create additional breeding sites with long water retention times.

Diversionary hosts: The presence of large numbers of domestic animals may reduce human biting rates. No information is available as to how the domestic animal population will be affected by the project.

Pesticides: The agricultural sector is planning intensive pesticide use on the rice crop. No information is available as to how this will affect vectors.

New vector species: The non-vector *Anopheles quadrannulatus* is extremely abundant. No information is available to determine whether vector or non-vector species will colonise the irrigation scheme.

Capability of health services and other protection agencies

Surveillance: National health statistics (see Handout) indicated considerable under-reporting of malaria cases. Statistics are always three years out-of-date. There is no information about localities in which malaria is particularly important. There are no statistical summaries available at health centre level. Many people do not attend government health centres when they have malaria, since they know that drugs are usually unavailable. Private doctors in town do not file case reports.

Vector control: Vector control is in response to emergencies. There is poor compliance with residual house spraying. Project managers are convinced of the importance of vector control but do not know how to reduce vector breeding through operation and maintenance. The farmers are not willing to maintain the irrigation ditches as they say that they have paid taxes for this purpose. Water tax paid by farmers is usually appropriated by central government so that operation and maintenance cannot be maintained at an optimal level.

Health centres: There are two health centres downstream of the project site with capacity for about 10,000 people. The staff have to hitchhike to town to collect their pay or request drug supplies and it seems unlikely that they will be able to cope with the extra requirements of a major construction site. The project planners have not held any discussions with the health sector and there is no provision for extra staff, buildings or drug supplies.

Summary of malaria risk

There is currently a high prevalence rate of malaria with seasonal transmission. The development project is expected to extend the transmission season and expose more people without adequate malaria control. The health risk is therefore high and increasing.

SCHISTOSOMIASIS

Urinary (*haematobium*) and intestinal (*mansoni*) forms are both present in San Serriffe. The prevalence rate is believed to be low in the project area. Animal reservoirs are not thought to be important. This is a "slow" disease which may not become a major community health problem during the first ten years of project operation.

Vulnerable communities

Very few of the Flong believe what they have been told about disease transmission. In all exposed communities children are seen as the major risk group because they like to bathe in reservoirs, irrigation systems and river pools. There are gender differences. Surveillance is restricted to schools.

Fishing folk: In the existing hydropower scheme the fishing folk who settled on the reservoir margin developed a high prevalence rate of infection after about seven years.

Farmers: The planned settlements are close to the night storage dams.

Farm labourers: Unplanned farm labourer settlements are expected to appear close to the irrigation ditches with no provision for water supply or sanitation.

Environmental factors

Night storage dams used for fishing and bathing favour large vector snail populations. The vector of intestinal schistosomiasis, *Biomphalaria pfeifferi*, thrives in stable, permanent water bodies but has a restricted distribution in San Serriffe. The vector of urinary schistosomiasis, *Bulinus globosus*, is more associated with unstable semi-permanent water bodies. The vectors are not usually found in rice fields.

Capability of health service and other protection agencies
Control currently depends exclusively on drugs such as praziquantel, which are very effective but relatively expensive. Stool and urine specimens are sometimes examined but knowledge of prevalence rates is based on occasional special surveys. The main objective of control is to identify the more heavily infected individuals and reduce morbidity. Urinary schistosomiasis is easier to detect because of the presence of blood in urine.

Summary of schistosomiasis risk
The increase in surface water suitable for snail breeding and the high exposure of children to contaminated waters is expected to produce an increasing prevalence and intensity of infection if no modifications are made to project plans.

SLEEPING SICKNESS

Cases of sleeping sickness are known in San Serriffe. There are reservoirs of infection in game animals.

Vulnerable community
This is an occupational disease of hunters and collectors such as poachers and loggers who are usually adult males. The growing shortage of firewood is forcing many women to forage further afield and it is not known whether they will come into contact with infected flies. The considerable economic disruption which will be experienced by communities displaced by the project is expected to make them more dependent on woodland produce and game animals. Some displaced families will move deeper into the bush.

Environmental factors
The tsetse fly vector, *Glossina morsitans*, is common in woodland wherever there is game or domestic animals. Tsetse control is only practised in some of the more important cattle ranching areas, north of Mount Flong. The distribution of reservoir game animals is now restricted to areas where access is difficult. Site surveyors reported seeing large herds of game upstream of the project site. Construction of access roads and a large reservoir will improve access to this hinterland.

Health service capability
Suspected cases of sleeping sickness are referred to large urban hospitals for full diagnosis and treatment.

Summary of sleeping sickness risk
The risk of sleeping sickness is low. However, an increase is expected if the disruption caused by the project leads to encroachment on the woodland reserve.

FILARIASIS AND DENGUE

These are largely urban/coastal diseases. Filariasis is a "slow" disease which affects mainly adults. Dengue is a "fast" disease which affects mainly children. Circulation of communities between project and towns will lead to importation of cases. Poor maintenance of project settlement sites will promote the breeding of the vectors. Displaced communities who join the urban drift and settle in slum areas will be at increased risk of infection.

GLOSSARY[1]

abscess	A cavity containing pus and surrounded by inflamed tissue.
acoustic trauma	Hearing loss, from exposure to continuous loud noise over a period of time or a sudden explosion or blow to the head or other injuries. May be temporary or permanent.
aflatoxicosis	A diseased condition caused by the presence of aflatoxins in the body.
aflatoxin	A class of mycotoxins produced by a mould that grows on damp food.
agro-chemicals	Chemicals used in the agricultural industry such as fertilizer, pesticides and weed killers.
AIDS	Auto Immune Deficiency Syndrome caused by infection with the human immunodeficiency virus.
airshed	A concept used to denote the boundaries of a mass of air. Often used in relation to pollution concentrations.
allergen	Any substance that induces an allergic reaction.
An.	Abbreviation of *Anopheles*.
anaemia	A condition characterized by a low haemoglobin level in the blood.
analysis	An examination in order to understand. *See* assessment.
anisakiasis	An infection of the gastrointestinal tract by larval nematodes of the subfamily Anisakidinae. People become infected by eating raw or inadequately treated fish.
Anopheline	One of two groups into which mosquitoes are divided.
Anopheles	A genus of mosquitoes that transmit malaria.
antenatal	A time period between conception and birth. It is important for women to have adequate treatment and advice during this time.
anthrax	A bacterial disease caused by the organism *Bacillus anthracis*.
antimony	A toxic chemical element.
appraisal	A critical examination of an identification report, which selects and ranks the various solutions from: points of relevance, technical, financial and institutional feasibility and socio-economic profitability and precedes the approval by the authorities of the proposed action.

---

[1] The definitions presented in this glossary are not official definitions. They have been formulated with a view to explaining technical terms to a non-technical readership. Some of the definitions have been obtained from the OECD *Methods and Procedures in Aid Evaluation* handbook.

aquatic	Living, growing or taking place in or on water.
arbovirus	An arthropod borne virus.
arsenic	A toxic chemical element.
arthritis	A condition characterized by painful and stiff joints that ultimately damages and deforms the joints involved producing considerable morbidity and disability.
arthropod	An animal group including insects, ticks and mites.
asbestos	A fine fibrous mineral that can damage the lungs.
asbestosis	A disease in which the lung tissue thickens in response to irritation by inhaled asbestos fibres and which consequently obstructs respiration.
Ascaris	A genus of large parasitic worms that infest the small and large intestines of humans and animals producing occasional symptoms. Also called roundworm. Found in temperate and tropical regions.
Asian tiger mosquito	Common name for *Aedes albopictus*.
assessment	An examination in order to decide. *See* analysis.
axil	The angle between the leaf and the stem. In some plants such as bromeliads water collection in the axil can provide breeding places for mosquitoes.
bacteria	A class of microscopic unicellular organisms that cause many diseases.
Bancroftian filariasis	Filariasis caused by the nematode *Wuchereria bancrofti*. See filariasis.
beedi	An indigenous Indian cigarette.
benefit-cost	A term that represents the relationship between the benefits accrued for the cost incurred.
benthic	Adjective of benthos.
benthos	Flora and fauna on the bottom of a water body.
benzene	A carcinogenic liquid, the fumes are irritating to the eyes, mucous membranes and upper respiratory tract and may cause dermatitis.
berm	An earthen bank raised above the ground.
bilharzia	See schistosomiasis.
biofuel	A biological, renewable source of energy.
biomass	Material derived from living matter.
biotopes	The smallest geographical unit of the biosphere or of a habitat that can be delimited by convenient boundaries and is characterised by its flora and fauna.
bivalves	A class of marine or freshwater molluscs.
blue-baby syndrome	A condition, suffered by babies, of insufficient

oxygen in the blood. It can be caused by nitrite ingestion.

bromeliads
: The family of plants to which the pineapple belongs. They are associated with breeding sites for mosquitoes.

bronchitis
: A disease in which the lining of the bronchial tubes of the lungs are inflamed. It may be caused by bacteria, viruses, chemicals and other substances such as asbestos and dusts.

bronchogenic carcinoma
: A malignant lung tumour that originates in the bronchi.

browse
: The shoots and leaves of plants. Fodder.

brucellosis
: A bacterial infection of animals causing abortion. It can be transmitted to man resulting in recurrent or chronic fever. Also called undulant fever.

Brugian filariasis
: Filariasis caused by *Brugia malayi. See* filariasis.

byssinosis
: A lung disease of cotton workers caused by an allergic reaction to dust or fungi in inhaled cotton, flax and hemp fibres.

cadmium
: A toxic element.

carcinogenic
: A substance that induces the development of cancer.

carcinoma
: A malignant, abnormal growth of new tissue.

carcinogenicity
: Of or pertaining to the ability to cause the development of a cancer.

cardiovascular
: Of or pertaining to the heart and blood vessels.

cassava
: Tapioca; an edible root. It contains toxic cyanide compounds in its skin and outer layers that need to be leached out during the cooking process.

Chagas
: A disease in South America affecting the heart, liver, spleen and colon due to infection with the parasite *Trypanosoma.*

checklist
: A list for verification purposes; a comprehensive list; an inventory.

chemoprophylaxis
: The use of antibiotics and chemicals to prevent the occurrence or spread of a disease in man.

chlorination
: A treatment process in which chlorine is used. For example, (1) to sterilise water or (2) to extract gold from ore.

chloroquine
: A drug used in the prophylaxis and treatment of malaria. There is increasing resistance in the malaria parasite to chloroquine.

cholera
: A highly infectious disease caused by *Vibrio cholerae* characterised by vomiting and rice water stools leading to rapid dehydration and death. It is spread by the faeco-oral route and

	contamination of water and food. It is subdivided into two biotypes, cholerae (classical) and El Tor.
chromium	A toxic element that can cause indolent and painful ulcers of the skin as well as dermatitis.
chromate	A salt of chromic acid that may be toxic.
chronic	Of a disease or disorder; developing slowly and persisting for a long time or constantly recurring.
coir	The strong fibre of coconut husks.
communicable disease	Any disease that is transmitted from a person or animal to another via a host of agents such as insects, foods and contaminated materials.
congenital	Dating from birth. Referring to a disease or deformity caused by defective or inoperative genes.
conjunctivitis	An inflammation of the thin transparent lining of the eye (the conjunctiva). It is caused by viruses, bacteria, chemical substances or degenerative changes.
cor pulmonale	An abnormal condition of the heart characterized by an enlarged right ventricle.
cortical cataract	An eye condition resulting in blurred and distorted vision.
cretinism	A disorder with physical and mental symptoms. Associated with iodine deficiency.
cross-resistance	The development of resistance to different antibiotics, drugs or pesticides of the same or related class by microorganisms or vectors.
Cryptosporidium	A microscopic organism normally found in the gut of animals. It is capable of producing diarrhoea in humans particularly in immuno-suppressed persons.
culvert	An arched channel beneath a road or railway to carry water.
cysticercosis	An infection with the larval stages of the pork tapeworm Taenia selium. It is acquired by eating inadequately cooked, infected pork.
DDT	An organochlorine based insecticide.
demographic	Relating to or pertaining to the study of populations; information about the composition and characteristics of a population.
dengue	An acute tropical fever caused by a virus, occasionally fatal; also known as break-bone fever. The vectors are mosquitoes of the Aedes genus.
dermatitis	An inflammation of the skin usually because of infection or irritation by chemical substances

that come in contact with the skin.

diarrhoea	Persistent purging or looseness of bowels commonly due to infection by microorganisms such as *Salmonella*.
dracunculiasis	A parasitic infection caused by infestation by the nematode *Dracunculus medinensis*. People are infected by drinking contaminated water. Also called guinea worm infection.
draught power	The use of animals to draw heavy loads.
drawdown	The magnitude of the change in water surface level in a well, reservoir or natural body of water resulting from the withdrawal of water.
dysentery	An inflammation of the large intestine associated with the frequent passage of bloody stools caused by *Entamoeba histolytica* (amoebic dysentery) and *Shigella* (bacillary dysentery) species.
dyspnoea	A shortness of breath. Difficulty in breathing.
ecology	The study of the relationship between communities of organisms and their environment.
effluent	Liquid industrial and agricultural waste; outflowing sewage during purification.
encephalitis	Inflammation of the brain tissue.
endemic	Of a disease or microorganism: indigenous to a geographic area or population.
enteric	Pertaining to the intestines; enteric fever or typhoid fever is an infectious disease caused by *Salmonella typhii* characterised by fever, rash, enlarged spleen and ulcers in the intestines.
epidemic	The occurrence in a community or region of cases of an illness, specific health-related behaviour, or other health-related events clearly in excess of normal expectancy within a specific area and time period.
epidemiology	The study of the distribution and determinants of health-related states or events in specified populations, and the application of this study to control of health problems.
epiphyte	A plant or animal growing or living on another plant or animal without being parasitic. (Adjective – epiphytic).
evaluation	An examination as systematic and objective as possible of an on-going or completed project or programme, its design, implementation and results with the aim of determining its: efficiency, effectiveness, impact, sustainability and relevance of the objectives with the

	purpose to guide decision-makers.
ex-post	Referring to an evaluation of an intervention after it has been completed with the aim to determine how well the aid has served its purposes and to draw conclusions for similar interventions in the future.
excreta	Faeces and urine.
farmers' lung	A respiratory disorder caused by inhalation of organic dusts from mouldy hay.
faeco-oral	Related to a route of transmission of pathogens that involves food, water or objects contaminated by faecal material entering the mouth.
falciparum malaria	The most severe form of malaria, caused by *Plasmodium falciparum*.
fallout	A deposit of dust from an explosion or industrial plant.
feasibility	A measure to prove that the technical options are sustainable and are also the best in that situation.
fertility	The ability to bear or reproduce.
filariasis	A disease caused by the presence of filarial worms in the blood and lymph nodes. The vector is a mosquito.
fluorosis	The condition resulting from excessive, prolonged ingestion of fluorine.
focus	Point or region of greatest activity of a disease and/or its vector. Plural – foci.
food security	Access to food for all people at all times, both physically and economically.
foraging	The act of searching for fodder for horses and cattle.
formaldehyde	A disinfectant, preservative and germicide. It is used to make synthetic resins. It is toxic.
fry	A swarm of young fish just spawned.
fuelwood	Wood collected for use as fuel.
fungi	Plants without chlorophyll which include mushrooms, and moulds.
fungicide	A chemical substance that kills fungi.
gastroenteritis	Inflammation of the lining of the stomach and intestines producing vomiting and diarrhoea caused by infection with microorganisms or toxins.
genotoxic	A substance which is toxic to genes.
geohelminth	A parasitic worm with part of its life cycle occurring in or on the soil.
genu valgum	A deformity in which the legs are curved inward so that the knees are close together, knocking as the person walks. Also called

knock-knee.

goitre	A condition in which the thyroid gland is abnormally enlarged, associated with iodine deficiency.
gonorrhoea	An infection of the genitourinary tract with the bacteria *Neisseria gonorrhoeae*. It is sexually transmitted.
grass-pea	A type of a legume, *Lathyrus sativus*, also called the chickling pea. Consumption can cause lathyrism. *See also* lathyrism.
groundwater	Water that occurs naturally beneath the ground surface and may include the fraction of the precipitation which infiltrates the land surface.
guinea worm	Common name for dracunculiasis.
habitat	The normal abode or locality of an animal or plant; the physical environment of a community; the place where a person or thing can usually be found.
haematuria	The presence of blood in the urine.
haemoglobin	The red oxygen-carrying pigment present in the red blood cell.
harbourage	A place of shelter and refuge; it may be natural or artificial.
hardware	Refers to mechanical equipment or infrastructure.
health hazard	A potential for causing harm to people.
health impact (of a development project)	A change in the frequency of some health indicators among the vulnerable community which is reasonably attributable to the project.
health risk	The possibility that a health hazard will cause harm to a human community. Measure of probability that a hazard will cause harm. As there are great uncertainties, only a simple ranking procedure can be used.
health risk management	Action intended to reduce health risk.
helminth	A parasitic worm.
hepatitis	An inflammatory condition of the liver which may be caused by bacterial, viral or parasitic infection, alcohol, drugs, toxins or transfusion of incompatible blood.
hepatitis A	A form of infectious viral hepatitis caused by the hepatitis A virus. It is spread by direct contact or through contaminated food and water.
hexachlorohexane	An insecticide of the organochloride (organic chemicals containing chloride) group.
hinterland	A region lying inland from a port or an urban centre, or a centre of affluence; terrain on the

	back of a folded mountain chain.
HIV	Human Immunodeficiency Virus that causes the Auto Immune Deficiency Syndrome (AIDS).
hookworm	A parasitic worm that causes anaemia.
host	An organism, on or in which a parasite lives and feeds.
hydatid disease	Infection with the larval stages of the dog tapeworm *Echinoccus granulosus*. Infection is acquired through faecal-oral contact and the larvae may migrate to any organ of the body.
hydraulic	Conveying water.
hydrogen sulphide	A gas that can cause asphyxiation.
hyperkeratosis	Thickening of the superficial layer of the skin.
hypoxia	Oxygen deficiency, may be caused by reduced oxygen carrying capacity, insufficient oxygen in inspired air, impaired tissue utilization of oxygen or inadequate blood flow.
HYV	High Yielding Variety, of agricultural crops.
immunization	A process that induces or increases the capacity of a person or animal to resist infection.
immuno-suppression	A decrease in the capacity of a person or animal to resist infection.
impact (of a development project)	A term indicating whether the project has had an effect on its surroundings in terms of: technical, economic, socio-cultural, health, institutional and environmental factors.
incidence	The number of cases of a specified disease diagnosed or reported during a defined period of time, divided by the number of persons in the population in which they occurred.
infectious	Of a disease organism, able to spread from one person to another.
infertility	The inability to bear or produce offspring.
influenza	An acute viral disease of the respiratory tract characterized by the presence of fever and severity of symptoms.
informal sector	Economic activities that are not subject to regulation.
inmigration	Migration inwards to a focal point.
Japanese Encephalitis	A mosquito borne arbovirus which can cause severe or fatal disease.
'jeepney'	A small bus characteristic of the Philippines.
jute	A plant fibre used for making sacks and mats.
keratitis	An inflammation of the cornea of the eye.
kwashiorkor	A nutritional disease of weaning children in

the tropics due to a relative deficiency of protein probably as a result of altered protein metabolism.

laryngeal	Of or pertaining to the larynx.
larynx	The upper part of the windpipe.
lathyrism	A disease caused by eating the grass-pea, *Lathyrus sativus*, which contains a toxic chemical substance. If it is consumed in large quantities the nerves in the spinal cord are damaged causing stiffness or paralysis of the lower limbs.
leachate	The products of leaching. *See* leaching.
leaching	The removal of readily soluble components, such as chlorides, sulphates and carbonates, from soil by percolating water.
Legionnaire's disease	An acute bacterial pneumonia caused by infection with *Legionella pneumophila*. Moist soil and contaminated air-conditioning cooling towers may be sources of organisms.
leishmaniasis	A disease caused by parasitic protozoa of the genus *Leishmania* that is transmitted from person to person by sandflies; also known as Kala-azar and Oriental sore.
leptospirosis	A disease caused by bacteria of the species *Leptospira*. It is transmitted to people by: contact with animals, moist soil, recreational, accidental or occupational immersion in water or vegetation contaminated with urine of infected animals such as pets and rodents.
leukaemia	Cancer of the blood.
listeriosis	An infectious disease caused by the bacteria *Listeria monocytogenes*.
loiasis	A form of filariasis caused by the worm *Loa loa*. It is transmitted by African deerfly or horsefly. It occurs in African moist forest.
lymphoma	Cancer of lymphoid tissue.
maloprim	A drug used in malaria prophylaxis.
malaria	A mosquito-borne disease caused by *Plasmodium* parasites. *See also falciparum* malaria and *vivax* malaria.
malnutrition	Undernourishment; a deficiency condition in which one or more necessary nutrients are unavailable in sufficient amounts for normal growth maintenance and health.
marginalization	The process by which a vulnerable population group is moved to the periphery of the socio-economic mainstream.

measles	An infectious viral disease common in children causing fever and a rash.
mefloquine	A drug used in the treatment of malaria, particularly chloroquine resistant malaria.
meningitis	An infection or inflammation of the membranes covering the brain and spinal cord.
meningococcal meningitis	Meningitis caused by the bacterium *Neisseria meningitidis.*
metastatic	Of or pertaining to the process by which tumour cells are spread to distant parts of the body.
methyl isocyanate	A highly reactive chemical which contains phosgene, a nerve gas.
methyl parathion	A relatively toxic pesticide.
micronutrient	A nutrient necessary for the normal growth and maintenance of the body but required in very small amounts, such as vitamins and minerals like iron and zinc.
migration	The permanent movement of a population from one habitat or location to another.
milch	Giving milk. Usually applied to cows which are kept for milking.
monitoring	A management function which uses a methodical collection of data to determine: whether the material and financial resources are sufficient, whether the people in charge have the necessary technical and personal qualifications; whether activities conform to work plans, and whether the work plan has been achieved and has produced the original objectives. *See* surveillance. <u>Environmental Monitoring:</u> observation of effects of development projects on environmental resources and values, including sampling and analysis, during construction and operation.
monocrotophos	A relatively toxic pesticide.
monoculture	The cultivation or culture of a single crop or species to the exclusion of others; as in replanting deforested areas with only one or few species.
morbidity	The condition of illness or abnormality; the rate at which an illness occurs in a particular area or population.
mortality	The condition of being subject to death; mortality rate (the death rate), the frequency or number of deaths in any specific region, age group, disease or other classification.
muco-cutaneous	Of or pertaining to the mucus membrane and skin.

mutagenic	Inducing genetic mutation(s) or increasing the mutation rate.
mutagenicity	Of or pertaining to the ability to cause genetic mutation.
mycotoxins	Toxins produced by fungi that are harmful.
nasal septum	The partition dividing the nostrils.
neonatal	Refers to the period from birth to 28 days of age.
neurotoxin	A toxin that has an affinity for the nervous system.
niacin	A member of the Vitamin B group of micronutrients.
nightsoil	A euphemism for human excreta stored in containers which are not connected to sewers. The containers are usually emptied at night and the partially decomposed matter may be used as a fertilizer.
nomadism	A sustainable lifestyle that requires frequent travelling from place to place usually within a well-defined geographical territory.
non-communicable	Cannot be spread from one person to another.
non-immune	Susceptible to a disease.
occupational disease	A disease common among workers engaged in a particular occupation brought about by the conditions of that occupation.
onchocerciasis	A disease caused by the parasitic worm *Onchocerca volvulus* that is transmitted by black flies; also called river blindness.
opencast	Relating to a mining process by which the material is excavated from an extensive area of the earth's surface.
Opisthorchis viverrini	A liver fluke acquired by eating inadequately cooked infected fish. Causes chronic liver disease and can be fatal.
organophosphorous	A group of chemicals used as pesticides.
outbreak	A sudden occurrence of, or increase in, cases of a disease in a population in an area or locality.
paludrine	A drug used in malaria prophylaxis.
paralytic shellfish poisoning	A toxic, neurologic condition that results from eating clams or mussels that have ingested protozoa containing the toxin saxitoxin.
parasite	An organism that lives on or in another organism termed the host, and draws nourishment from it. (Adjective – parasitic)
parathion	An insecticide from the organophosphate group of insecticides.

particulate	Having the form of particles.
pastoralism	The keeping of herds of cattle, goats, sheep or similar animals.
pathogen	An organism that causes disease. Most pathogens are microscopic in size.
periurban	Relating to localities bordering a city or other urban area.
phosgene	A suffocating and highly poisonous gas.
phosphine	1. Hydrogen phosphide, a toxic gas. 2. A coal tar dye, extremely destructive to some lifeforms.
plague	A disease caused by infection with the bacillus *Yersinia pestis* that is usually transmitted from rodents to people by fleas.
plume	A narrow column of smoke or noxious gases.
pneumoconiosis	A disease of the lung caused by long-term inhalation of dust, usually mineral dusts of occupational or environmental origin.
pneumonia	An inflammation of the lung caused by pathogenic organisms such as bacteria, viruses and chemicals.
poliomyelitis	A communicable disease caused by one of the three polio viruses that may result in paralysis.
potable water	Water that is palatable and safe for human consumption; in which any toxic substances, pathogenic organisms and factors have been reduced to safe or acceptable levels.
prevalence	The number of people ill because of a particular disease at a particular time in a given population. Often expressed as a rate.
prophylaxis	The methods used to prevent the occurrence of, or progression to disease.
protection agency	A government agency responsible for protecting the health and safety of the community and the environment.
protein-energy	Energy derived from the metabolism of proteins in the human body.
psittacosis	A type of pneumonia that is transmitted from birds to humans.
pulmonary	Of or pertaining to the lungs or the respiratory system.
pyrethroid	A group of powerful synthetic insecticides.
pyrethrum	A natural insecticide extracted from chrysanthemum flowers.
q fever	An acute febrile illness, usually respiratory, caused by *Coxiella burnetii*. Humans acquire the disease through contact with infected animals by inhalation (from hides), consuming infected milk or tick bite.

recrudescence	The recurrence of a disease because of reinfection rather than a reactivation of existing microorganisms.
resistance	The capacity by an organism to remain unaffected by toxins or pathogenic microorganisms.
respiratory	Pertaining to the lungs and the breathing apparatus of the body.
Rhodamine B dye	A bright red colouring agent.
rodenticide	A chemical used to kill rodents.
roundworm	A group of parasitic worms including *Ascaris* and *Strongyloides*.
runoff	Precipitation which flows over the surface of the land as opposed to that which penetrates beneath the surface.
Salmonella	Bacteria that cause typhoid, diarrhoea and other diseases. It is usually associated with poultry and animal husbandry and transmitted from animal to humans and from humans to humans by the faecal-oral route and contamination of food and drinking water.
sandfly	A common name for flies of the group phlebotomine including the genus *Phlebotomus*. Sometimes vectors of leishmaniasis.
scabies	A contagious disease caused by the mite *Sarcoptes scabiei* which burrows in the outer layers of skin. It is transmitted by skin contact.
Schistosoma haematobium	A species of *Schistosoma* found chiefly in Africa and the Middle East. Affects the bladder and pelvic organs causing painful, frequent and bloody urination.
Schistosoma japonicum	A species of *Schistosoma* found in Japan, The Philippines and Eastern Asia. Causes gastrointestinal ulcerations and fibrosis of the liver.
Schistosoma mansoni	A species of *Schistosoma* which is found in Africa, the Middle East, the Caribbean and South America. Causes symptoms similar to *Schistosoma japonicum*.
schistosomiasis	A disease, caused by infestation of the human body by the worms of *Schistosoma*, characterised by the passing of blood in the urine or stool. Also called bilharzia.
scoping	A process of defining which communities, hazards, geographical areas and project phases to include in an impact assessment.
screening	A process of sorting project proposals as part of an initial environmental examination to

	ascertain the need for health impact assessment.
scrub typhus	Mite-borne typhus fever.
seasonality	Showing periodicity related to seasons.
sedentarization	The settlement of nomads in permanent locations.
septicaemia	Systemic infection of the blood stream.
septic fringe	The unsanitary environment of slums and squatters.
seropositive	A positive reaction in a blood test.
sewage	Human excreta and wastewater flushed along a sewer pipe.
Shigella	A genus of pathogenic bacteria that causes gastroenteritis and bacterial dysentery. *See* dysentery.
silicosis	A chronic lung disease caused by long-term inhalation of silica dust.
Simulium damnosum	A species of biting fly that are vectors of onchocerciasis (river blindness). Found near fast flowing water. Common name is blackfly.
smallholder	A farmer who owns or rents a small area of farmland.
soakpit	A pit to promote seepage of effluent into the ground.
software	The rules by which hardware is effectively managed.
spillway	A structure for the discharge of overflow water.
standpipe	A tap on the end of a free standing water pipe.
steppe	A dry, grassy, generally treeless and uncultivated plain.
subsistence	Providing the bare necessities of living.
sullage	Domestic dirty water not containing excreta; also called grey water.
surveillance	A continuing scrutiny of all aspects of the occurrence and spread of a disease that are pertinent to effective control. Alternatively, a special reporting system for a particular health problem for a limited time period.
susceptibility	The incapacity to resist contracting a disease when exposed to the agent causing that disease.
sustainability	The extent to which the objectives of an aid activity will continue after the project assistance is over; the extent to which the groups affected by the aid want to take charge themselves to continue accomplishing its objectives.
syndrome	A characteristic pattern of symptoms and signs that describe a disease entity.
synergistic	Pertaining to a combined or co-ordinated

action in which the effect of a substance or an organ is augmented by the use with another.

tailings	Soil and other debris washed out of a mine works.
tannin	A chemical used in tanning and dying.
tapeworm	A parasitic worm that infects humans and animals.
teratogenicity	Refers to the ability to cause interference with normal prenatal development in the foetus.
tilapia	A group of edible freshwater fish.
'top-down'	Refers to a theory in development in which improvements and incentives are envisaged to percolate through the society and economy from the top level to the broad based lower levels.
transmission	Any route by which a human being is exposed to an infectious agent.
trichinosis	A disease caused by the migration through the skin of larvae of a worm called *Trichinella spiralis*.
Trichuris	A parasitic worm that infests the intestines of humans.
trypanosomiasis	A disease of animals and humans caused by a *Trypanosoma* parasite; called sleeping sickness in Africa and Chagas disease in South America.
tsetse	A blood-sucking fly that is the vector of trypanosomiasis in Africa.
tuberculosis	A chronic and disabling disease of the lungs, and less frequently other parts of the body, which is fatal if not treated.
tungsten	Wolfram. A rare metal.
typhoid	An infectious disease in humans caused by *Salmonella typhii* bacteria. It is transmitted by the faeco-oral route and contamination of drinking water and food.
typhus	An infectious disease spread from person to person by the body louse, fleas, mites or ticks. Caused by microorganisms of the genus *Rickettsia*.
uranium	A radioactive metal.
vector	An animal – often an insect – transmitting an infection from person to person or from infected animals.
Vivax malaria	A form of malaria caused by *Plasmodium vivax*. It is the most common form of malaria and rarely fatal. *See also* malaria.

vulnerability   The liability to be injured or damaged or hurt.

watershed   A ground area (usually elevated) either side of which rainfall flows into different river systems. In the US the term is used to denote a rainfall catchment area for a river system.

whipworm   Common name for the parasitic roundworm *Trichuris trichiura*. Infects the intestinal tract. Indirectly transmitted from human to human through soil.

wild food   Food which is gathered, fished, or hunted, but not cultivated.

zoonosis   An infectious disease transmissible under natural conditions from animals to humans.

zooprophylaxis   The use of animals to divert vectors from humans.

INDEX